1

# Table of Contents

# Introduction

A phlebotomy technician, also called a phlebotomist, is an integral healthcare worker of the medical laboratory team whose main function is the collection of blood samples from patients by microtechniques or venipuncture. The phlebotomy technician collects and transports laboratory specimens, and is the patient's primary contact with the laboratory. The technician must assure patient safety and quality of care, and certification mandates strict professional behavior and the standards of practice for phlebotomists.

**Job Duties**

Phlebotomy technicians also are involved with patient data entry. They have to work well under pressure and communicate effectively with others, as well as help the patient remain calm during the venipuncture or blood collection process. Safety precautions are taken for the prevention of infectious disease transmission. Various job duties of the phlebotomy technician may include:

- Draw blood from donors in hospitals, blood banks, and other similar medical facilities

- Obtain blood from patients in the doctor's office, hospital, or laboratory setting

- Assemble necessary laboratory equipment, such as blood collection devices, needles, gauze, alcohol swabs, and tourniquets

- Verify records, and maintain patient or donor information

- Label and store blood for processing

- Conduct a patient interview

- Test blood samples

- Screen donors at the blood bank

- Assess vital signs

**Education and Training**

A phlebotomy technician must have a high school diploma or GED, with training and documented education. Phlebotomy technician programs are available at many career colleges, online, and accredited schools. Phlebotomy training courses vary in length and typically lead to a certificate of completion or a diploma.

## Certification and Licensure

The test to certify is called the Certified Phlebotomy Technician (CPT) examination, and the fee is $150. Each state decides licensure, but most do not require this. Employers prefer to hire experienced employees who have certification and/or a license. This indicates that the technician has passed a national examination and meets certain standards of competence.

The Phlebotomy Technician Certification (CPT) program is accredited by the National Commission for Certifying Agencies (NCCA), which issues CPT certifications through the National Healthcareer Association (NHA).

# Patient Preparation

## Preparing the Patient

The first section of the certified phlebotomy technician (CPT) review course covers the patient preparation techniques, which are required prior to providing patient care. Patient preparation involves providing an introduction to the patient, explaining the procedure, reviewing requisition, receiving implied and informed consent, identifying the patient, determining the appropriate sample, selecting the site, applying the appropriate antiseptic, and verifying the patient complies with the appropriate testing requirements, such as fasting or medication. The guidelines are set in place to ensure that the patient gets the information needed. These guidelines help employers avoid civil action that could occur.

While explaining the process and receiving compliance from the patient is an important part of proper patient care, the patient must also be greeted with a certain personal approach to establish a professional relationship. This includes:

- Dressing in a manner that portrays your appearance as well-kept.

- Maintaining good eye contact with the patient prior to starting the procedure.

- Allowing the patient to have personal space and a comfortable level of contact prior to explaining the procedure.

- Answering any questions.

### Introduction to the Patient

Prior to any type of testing, the phlebotomist should provide an introduction based upon the type of testing that will be done. This is accomplished by greeting the patient, providing them with basic information regarding the test, and then answering any questions they may have with the correct answers. After the answer has been provided to the patient, the patient must be allowed to ask additional questions, until the questions have been answered in a clear and concise manner. This ensures that the patient feels well-informed and completely comfortable by having all of their questions answered.

The information provided to the patient is given through oral communication, or the patient can be provided with a pamphlet, which gives information on the testing process and answers any additional questions. After allowing the patient to look over the information in the provided packet, the phlebotomist should ask the patient if he or she has any questions about the information before moving onto the next step of patient preparation.

Be sure to identify yourself to the patient by using your first name, and then explain to the patient that your intent is to draw blood that will be used for testing. When speaking with the patient, all information you provide must be in an easily understood manner. Without knowledge of medical practice and the different techniques involved, medical jargon can be difficult to understand for patients. An explanation of all information must be provided without using medical terminology, and the patient should be asked if he or she understands the information prior to moving onto the next question. Talk with the patient in a manner that acknowledges the different needs. Also, when you are explaining the procedure to the patient, you may want to explain your duty as a phlebotomy technician prior to explaining the testing process.


**Explaining the Phlebotomy Procedure**

Prior to starting any type of testing process, the phlebotomy technician must explain the test to the patient. This includes telling the patient that you are planning to draw blood, the location where the blood will be drawn, how much blood will be drawn from the testing site, and what will be done with the blood once it has been drawn. A full explanation of the steps should be given prior to having the patient sign a consent form.

Solid communication is a main factor during the testing process as well. It is important that all communication, both verbal and non-verbal, is done on a basis that takes into consideration the *right amount* of information. For example, telling the patient you will be drawing blood may not be enough information - it is best to explain that you will be using a needle to take blood from a specific location, which will then be captured into a tube and sent out for testing. This ensures that the patient has a complete understanding of the testing process.


**Communicating with the Patient**

Good communication with the patient is based upon different actions, which include:

- Eye contact

- Good posture

- Well-groomed appearance

- Respecting personal space

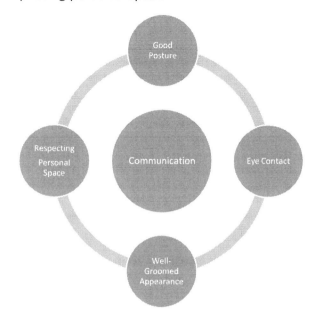

## Negative Communication

To avoid negative communication, you should avoid:

- Drooping shoulders

- Holding held down

- Avoiding eye contact

- Wearing too much jewelry

- Invading personal space (getting too close prior to introducing yourself)

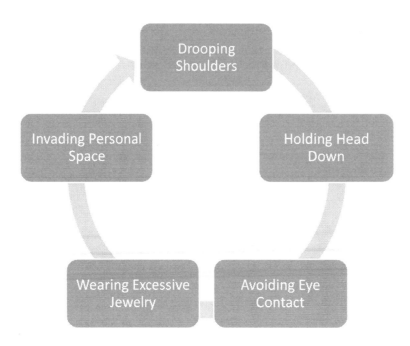

## Active Listening

Active listening is another important aspect of explaining the procedure. After you have explained everything involved with the testing process, you must take the time to listen to the patient and give your full level of attention. By providing the patient with attention, you can ensure that you are able to answer the questions they have regarding the procedure to the best of your ability.

## The Patient Care Partnership Act

Although not legally binding, the Patient Care Partnership Act states that taking these communication steps will ensure the patient receives the highest quality of care possible. The patient has the right to receive information on all testing procedures, a clean, safe environment, and involvement of care and protection of the privacy before and during the care provided.

## Ethics and Duty of Care

A professional appearance and attitude is the most important aspect of the patient preparation process. Professionalism at the work place is considered to be the behavior, appearance, and qualities that characterize a professional person. These qualities are set forth in the ethics system, and involve a strict ethical code of contact between the patient and the medical professional who is providing the patient with care.

The phlebotomy technician has a responsibility of fulfilling the "Duty of Care" rights that all patients have, before and during the testing process. According to these standards, the previous and following standards ensure that the patient does not experience infringement, slander, or libel, which can result in legal action. While these could affect the reputation of the individual who is receiving care, they are each different acts that affect the patient. Damage could occur to the patient's reputation, the level of care through improper communication, wrongful documentation of the information received, or allowing information regarding a patient to be received by someone who isn't involved directly within the patients care.

## Consent Forms

In order for the patient to make an informed decision regarding the care they receive from the phlebotomy technician, he or she must fully understand all information given by providing a consent form. The patient should fully understand:

- Any risks associated with the testing process.

- The benefits that will be received by testing.

- If the tests are part of the patient's healthcare needs, for research purposes, or part of a study.

- What he or she can learn about health status based upon the testing.

- How the testing process may affect quality of life.

- What is necessary once he or she leaves the testing facility after the specimen is collected and any additional testing requirements are met.

## Testing Requirements

For cases where special testing requirements were set forth, it is important that the phlebotomy technician ensures the patient has met these specifications prior to performing the test. This means you will need to ask questions regarding the testing requirements. An example of this would be inquiring about the last time the patient had anything to eat or drink prior to the test. By ensuring the patient has met the testing requirements, the test can be completed, and the results of the test will be accurate.

Upon receiving information that the testing requirements were fully met, the first form of patient identification should be addressed. This may include asking the patient to state his or her full name to you prior to moving forward with further patient preparation. One of the most common acts of legal action filed against a phlebotomy technician is due to lack of proper patient identification and improper methods of testing

### Receiving Implied or Informed Consent

Prior to performing the blood testing, the patient must provide both written and oral consent. This is done in the form of signing a contract read by the patient, which further explains the testing process, requirements of the testing process, and the standards set in place for the patient. Once this paper is signed by the patient, and dated with the correct date, the person who stands witness to the consent must also sign and date the paper. This protects all parties prior to the testing process, and ensures that all information about the process has been fully explained to the patient through verbal and written information.

After the patient is given the written consent, a verbal consent is also needed to go ahead and start the testing process. This is done by asking the patient if they completely understand all of the information that has been provided to them, and then having the patient answer the question with a yes. Once both of these consents are received, the testing process can begin. However, according to the standards set in place for safe testing practices prior to the procedure, the testing process cannot be carried out without both of these consents, and one form of identification must be viewed prior to the blood draw.

### Denying Consent

The patient has the right to deny agreement with the consent that you have provided to him or her. This can be done in two different ways:

- The patient may deny signing the consent form, which is provided to them by the facility. Without written consent, the work cannot be performed on the patient.

- Even if the consent form is signed, the patient must also provide a verbal consent prior to having the test done. If the patient refuses to acknowledge the phlebotomy technician during the oral portion of the consent, then the technician cannot proceed. Examples include placing the arm up for the blood work, while paying attention to things going on around them and not to the information they are being asked. This is considered to be a denial of consent from the patient, and the testing process cannot be completed until the patient acknowledges the phlebotomy technician and gives oral consent.

**Minors, Guardians, and Caregivers**

If the patient is under the age of 18, the oral and written consent process must be completed by their legal guardian or parent. Proof of identification must be obtained by the person who is providing the consent for the minor, and a copy of the identification card should be made and stored within the patient file.

When receiving consent from a legal guardian of a minor patient, all medical history involving the patient must be reviewed with the caregiver in order to ensure the information that is on file is correct. Any changes that need to be made must be documented, along with the previous information available during the review of the medical history. The information reviewed during this time should include:

- Previous allergies the patient may have

- Past illnesses, past hospital stays, any surgeries the patient had

- Medications the patient is taking

- The admission requirements that are set in place for the patient based upon the health care plan that they have

While a patient of legal age can provide this type of information to the phlebotomy technician, anyone who is signing is required to provide the information needed for the phlebotomy technician to move forward with care. This type of process is also used for those who cannot discuss their condition without the help of a caregiver, such as an elderly individual who is experiencing issues with memory or someone whose health affects his or her ability to provide clear and concise answers based on their previous medical history.

One of the main reasons why legal action is taken against a medical company is because the proper consent was not received by the patient. By having a written consent, a witness, and an oral consent on file, the medical professionals working to provide patient care can protect themselves from any legal action, should the patient claim that they did not receive the information necessary or provide consent to perform the collection process. The written portion of the consent form will be scanned, stored within the computer, and a copy will also be kept within the patient file for future reference.

## Positively Identifying the Patient

Set forth as one of the most crucial aspects of the testing process, positively identifying the patient is done through a variety of steps that all must be taken properly. In order to properly identify the patient, the National Patient Safety Goals established by the Joint Commission on Accreditation of Healthcare Organizations (JCAHO), recommended that at least two forms of patient identification be used prior to testing. These forms can vary based upon the location of testing, but should include two of the following:

- Photo identification card
- Matching patient I.D. bracelet with order form
- Checking patient room number with corresponding I.D tag
- Receiving personal information via oral communication, such as birthdate

Properly identifying the patient is a three-step process, which must be fully completed prior to performing any type of testing procedure. For acute care settings, the patient I.D tag must be checked upon entering the room, and then the testing I.D. number must be matched with the number that is found on the order form. This process includes three steps: validate, compare, and ask. The phlebotomy technician can eliminate error or miscommunication by meeting each of these steps properly.

## Eliminating Errors

The National Patient Safety Goals states that errors in the testing process by providing the wrong patient with testing can be completely eliminated. If there is any type of error or miscommunication during this time, further investigation must be completed to ensure the patient proper identity prior to testing. The patient must be asked to state full name and date of birth, which must match will the information that is present on the testing sheet. The additional steps that are needed include:

- Meeting with hospital staff to view the photo I.D card that was presented by the patient prior to being admitted into the facility, or
- Meeting with a family member of the patient and having them identify the patient prior to performing the test.

For outpatient settings, a photo identification card must be presented by the patient, and a copy of the identification card must be made and attached to the patient's file. Taking blood from the wrong patient is considered to be patient negligence, and will result in punishment and the possibility of legal action if the patient files legal suit.

While working towards properly identifying the patient, there are certain things that must be avoided in ordered to consider the information obtained proper and right. Do not call the patient by their first name. Certain patients may not be in the right mental state during the time of testing, and they may repeat the name that they are called, even if this is not their name.

Do not start the testing process without first looking at the information provided, receiving the patient's identifying information, and then comparing the information that was provided with the information you have on the testing slip provided by the physician.

Prior to starting the testing, you must determine the proper location for the sample to be drawn from. The patient should be placed in a position that allows access to all antecubital veins. It is recommended that the site where the sample is taken from is near the bicep area. However, there are certain situations where the blood should not be taken from a specific location.

Once you have found the location where you plan to draw the blood from, a tourniquet must be wrapped around the area, and the veins within that area must be probed with your hand in order to ensure that the testing site is appropriate. While the medial cubital, cephalic, and basilic veins are the most preferred sites, the testing may also be done in the dorsal hand veins.

Once the testing site has been properly determined, you can remove the tourniquet from the area, and then begin preparing the testing materials. Do not leave the tourniquet on while preparing the materials.

### Selecting a Site that Minimizes Patient Risk

Certain conditions and situations can put the patient at risk if testing is done on a particular area of the body. In order to minimize the patient's risk, several factors need to be taken into consideration prior to testing, even when a good location for the testing sample to be obtained has been determined.

*Areas to Avoid*

- Scarred, bruised, and/or swollen areas
- Those near an IV site
- Where previous blood sample testing was performed and not fully healed
- The feet and ankles (unless otherwise directed due to certain special condition circumstances that can occur)
- Where a radical mastectomy is present, such as the left arm

If a patient seems agitated or hostile, it is important to get help from another staff member prior to testing in order to avoid injuring the patient. There are tendons and ligaments that are easily mistaken as veins. By asking the patient to open and close their fist, while checking these areas, you can determine if it is a vein you are planning to test.

Many Americans have an intense fear of needles. In this type of situation, the fear may cause the patient to experience several negative effects of testing. This can include fainting, breathing attacks, and convulsions. There have been 23 reported incidents of death related to this intense fear. In this type of situation, it is important that steps are taken prior to administering the blood work, which will ensure that the patient is calm and safe while they have the process of collecting a sample completed.

### Determining Site Accessibility

The patient's current condition and age play a large role in determining the proper site of sample testing. For older patients, certain areas may be difficult for testing, and the skin in that area may be thin, thus resulting in damage to the area when venipuncture occurs. If the patient is in critical condition, injured, or has an illness, certain areas of the body must be avoided while determining the proper site for testing.

By taking age and condition into consideration, the proper type of testing can be determined. There are two types of methods available for drawing blood from the patient. These types include venipuncture and dermal. While they both serve the same purpose, and allow the phlebotomist to collect the specimen that is needed, the tests have varying results.

### Dermal Method

The dermal method requires less of a puncture to take place, thus it is not as important that the patient sit completely still during the testing process. The risk of injuring the patient is lowered greatly when this type of testing process is used, because the needle that punctures the skin is immediately retracted once the puncture takes place. However, due to the method of collection, the testing process takes longer to complete, and could actually pose a greater risk to people within a certain category.

The risk of oxygen meeting with the blood is greater during this type of collection process, and the delayed collection speed can result in blood clotting while it is being taken from the site, and also having the blood produce a faulty result when sent to the lab. The amount of blood needed with this test is much less than that required for a venipuncture test. This is an important factor to consider when the testing is done on people who cannot afford to lose a lot of blood, such as infants and those with blood loss due to trauma.

For testing that takes longer to complete once sent to the lab, the dermal collection method should generally be avoided as the specimen does not stay fresh as long as it would with the standard method of withdrawal.

## Venipuncture Method

While the risk of injury is greater with the venipuncture collection method, this type of draw can collect large amounts of blood very quickly, and the specimen will be preserved for a greater period, resulting in test results that are more accurate. This type of testing process punctures deep into the vein, and then the needle is kept inside of the vein the entire time the blood is being drawn from the site.

When the proper injection site is not determined by considering all aspects involving the patients current age and condition, there are certain risks present. Hitting a nerve within the area of puncture is one issue that can occur without the proper assessment. When this occurs, they are will be damaged permanently, and it can experience a significant amount of pain.

## Aseptic Technique

In order to prevent infection from occurring during the collection of the blood specimen, site must be properly cleaned with the right agents. The agents used for cleaning the skin are designed to remove any type of bacteria present on the skin, as well as to eliminate the risk of the bacteria entering the skin during the puncture, which can cause an infection.

The most common form of antiseptic used is rubbing alcohol, which is applied to the site in a specialized manner. While alcohol is generally used to cleanse the area, some patients may have an allergy to this substance. A phlebotomist must make it routine to ask the patient if they are allergic to the cleansing agent used in order to prevent the risk of a reaction.

If an allergy is present, there are alternative antiseptic agents available to cleanse the skin prior to performing the testing process. The most common type agent used for cleaning the skin (if alcohol cannot be used) is povidone iodine. Regardless of the agent used, there is a specialized method of application that must be followed with all agents in order to properly cleanse the area and ensure that the risk of infection is reduced.

*Steps of Skin Sanitizing*

1. All materials should be prepared for the testing process prior to cleaning the testing area in order to eliminate the risk of infection

2. Use a circular motion when cleansing the area

3. Start from the direct location of entry when cleaning with the agent, and then work your way out in a two- to three-inch radius around the testing site.

4. Be sure to clean all areas around the testing site with the solution, as well. Bacteria can spread rather quickly, and by only cleaning the area where insertion will take place, the risk of infection is greater

5. After cleaning the area, allow it to air dry completely prior to inserting the needle and collecting the specimen. By inserting the needle before the area has completely dried, the chemical can enter the skin where the insertion takes place, and the agent can affect the blood and cause irritation

6. Once the area has dried, immediately apply to tourniquet to the testing area and start the process

**Verifying Patient Compliance with Testing Requirements**

In order for the test to be accurate, there are certain requirements set forth for the patient. These must be assessed when explaining the procedure and again right before taking the specimen. All information received from the patient should be documented, and in certain cases where special standards are set in place, the testing process may need to be scheduled for another date, such as if the patient did not meet fasting needs, which would produce a faulty result.

It is important that the patient agrees with these standards prior to the testing, and he or she must provide you with an oral agreement that they have information on the requirements, agree to these, and meet all of the standards set in place for them prior to the test. All information collected during this time must be sent along with the specimen, including the last time the patient had anything to eat or drink prior to the test.

Prior to collecting the specimen, some patients will need to have certain medical states checked. This can include:

- Taking the patient's blood pressure

- Taking the patient's basal temperature

- Listing all medications that the patient is currently taking

In order to ensure that the patient meets the requirements set forth for the testing process, the physician will generally provide a written guide that explains the requirements of the test, such as how long the patient must fast prior to the blood sample collection. You should ask if this information was provided to the patient by the physician, as well as if he or she had complied with the information. Explaining the importance of complying with the directions in order to receive accurate results will help the patient to understand why taking certain steps is essential for proper testing, and this will help to simplify future testing processes.

# The Collection Process

The primary role of a phlebotomy technician is to collect blood specimens in a manner that is safe for the patient, protects the individual drawing the blood, and also works to meet all of the requirements, while also performing the task in the most cost-efficient manner. There are several steps involved in collecting the blood sample, and all of these steps must be completed exactly as stated in order to meet all standards.

These are the steps:

- Proper insertion and removal of the needle used for testing
- Choosing the best collection method based on patient age and condition
- Ensuring patient safety during the collection process
- Performing the testing process in the correct order
- Recognizing common complications that can occur during the testing process
- Identifying patient signs that can pose an issue during the testing process
- Following the proper order of withdraw during a venipuncture process
- Following the proper order of steps during a capillary collection
- Ensuring that the tubes used for collection the specimen meet the requirements
- Properly assembling the equipment needed for the collection
- Using evacuated tubes for collection after the testing process
- Verifying that the equipment used during the testing process is high quality

## Venipuncture Collection

The order of steps regarding the venipuncture procedure refers to the method of retrieval used while obtaining the specimen from the patient. By properly applying these methods when performing the venipuncture, the risk of analytical errors and patient complications can be avoided. The process of properly performing the venipuncture involves completing all steps involved in the correct manner. The steps involved include ordering, drawing, labeling, collecting, handling, and collecting the blood specimen.

## Collecting Supplies

Obtain the proper lab collecting trays. Refer to the office policy set in place for proper tray handling. The tray used for the method of collection must be lightweight, easy to handle, and have enough space on it to handle all of the materials.

- Collect both latex and non-latex gloves for the testing. The gloves used for testing must meet the standards set forth in the OSHA guidelines.

- Gather the hubs needed for drawing the specimen. The hubs may have a vacuum feature, and they are for single use collection only. If the collection must be transferred to a new container, the use of special transfer hubs is available.

- Obtain the needle of appropriate gauge for the blood collection.

- Use a sterile syringe. The syringe that is used should be in the original packaging. If the syringe has been removed from the packaging prior to the testing, it is no longer considered to be sterile and should be disposed of.

- Blood collection tubes should be obtained based upon the types of testing necessary during the retrieval.

- The appropriate cleansing agent should be placed on the tray for use prior to the insertion of the needle. An alcohol pad and the alternative should be readily available.

- Supplies for after testing should be obtained. This includes gauze and bandages.

- Ice and a warming device must be present on the tray

- The specimen collection manual should be available for reference if a question should arise during the collection process.

## Assembling Supplies

When you are preparing the supplies for the patient, they must all be taken out of the original packaging in front of the patient who is receiving the treatment. All equipment must be set up in a manner that meets the guidelines in place. The syringes must have all safety features activated prior to attaching them to the tubes that will collect the specimen.

## Tourniquet Application

The tourniquet will need to be applied to the arm prior to collecting the specimen. This is done by wrapping the band tight enough above the area of collection that it allows the vein to properly display, so the needle can be inserted into the area as easily as possible. This should not be left on the arm for more than two minutes at a time, and the process of inserting the needle and collecting the blood should start as soon as the tourniquet is attached.

## Prioritizing the Retrievals

When you are collecting multiple samples, you must prioritize the sample retrievals prior to starting the testing.

- STAT testing means the specimen must be collected right away.

- URGENT means the sample should be collected as soon as possible.

- STANDARD means the collection should be done in when possible, and there is no rush on this type of collection.

## Performing the Venipuncture

1. The patient's identity must be determined prior to inserting the needle for collection.

2. The appropriate method of collection must be determined by the technician. While the vein is the preferred method of withdraw in many cases, special conditions may require the use of capillary collection.

3. Sanitize the hands using the correct methods, and then put on the protective gear needed to protect both you and the patient during the retrieval method, such as gloves and a face mask.

4. Position the patient carefully, in a manner that allows you to have direct eye contact with the site where the work is performed.

5. Apply the tourniquet to the arm, three to four inches below the bicep if the blood is being drawn at this site. For other areas, the tourniquet should still be applied about the same distance from the site of retrieval.

6. If the vein is not visible after putting the tourniquet on the arm, the patient should be asked to make a fist, which will make the vein visible.

7. Apply a cleaning agent to the skin in the correct manner set forth in the standards of application. This manner includes applying the alcohol pad that contains the fluid to the area in a circular motion, which includes the site where the needle will enter the skin, as well as a radius around the testing site of two to three inches.

8. Using the hand, grasp the patients arm firmly, and then stretch the area of the skin where the insertion will take place. Be sure to use the thumb when completing this step, as this will ensure that the skin is not stretched too far, which can result in an injury to the skin where the needle is inserted.

9. Once the skin is taut, insert the needle through the skin and into the lumen of the vein, at a 15 to 30 degree angle.

10. Check to ensure that the blood is properly flowing from the vein within the arm, through the needle, and into the collection tube.

**After the Venipuncture**

1. After the specimen has been collected from the patient, leave the needle in the vein, and remove the tourniquet if it is still on the testing site.

2. Apply a gauze pad to the area where the needle is inserted.

3. Once the needle has been covered by a piece of gauze, you can activate the safety device located on the needle. This device works to retract the needle from the skin.  After it has retracted, cover the needle with protective material.

4.  Ask the patient to hold the gauze in place with pressure on the testing site, while you take the steps needed to dispose of the materials used during the collection process.

5. Once the materials have been disposed of properly, you must immediately mark all of the collected specimens with the appropriate label. Any materials that contain blood or body fluids are considered to be a hazard to health, thus disposing of these materials in accordance with OSHA standards is important to ensure the patient receives the highest level of care, and all other personnel within the building are protected from health risks during the testing process. This application of labels must be done prior to returning to the patient.

6. Examine the puncture to ensure bleeding has slowed. If so, put the gauze in place, and then cover it with a bandage in order to supply the area with the pressure needed to stop the bleeding completely.

7. The pressure applied by the gauze and the bandage will stop the bleeding quickly by allowing the blood to clot. The patient should be instructed to remove the gauze from the area of withdrawal 5 to 10 minutes after it was applied.

**Completing the Process**

Any liquid that leaks from the testing equipment must be cleaned before any additional steps can be taken. The medical professionals working at the lab or hospital must work as a team, and another team member should be called upon to clean up the waste. The Environmental Protection Agency (EPA) states that any material that leaks during the process should be cleaned from the area with a 1:10 bleach solution or another cleaning solution that is approved by the EPA.

Capillary collection of a blood specimen is done by puncturing the dermis of the skin, and then collecting the blood located under this area. This method of collection is preferred for some, based on the patient's age and certain medical conditions, because it allows the blood to be collected without entering a vein.

The blood collected during the capillary collection method contains material from the patient arterioles, venues, and capillaries. It will also include interstitial and intracellular fluids. Due to the process of collection that is used, a much smaller amount of blood is needed for the test. Unlike blood that is taken from the vein, the capillary collection method is more difficult and requires a precise collection method.

The capillary collection method is generally suggested when drawing blood from a newborn baby. When testing is done on a newborn, using the heel of the foot is recommended. The heel can be used until the child is of one year of age, then the process should be done on the patients finger. When the procedure is performed correctly, the stick used to puncture the skin and collect the specimen can work within these areas without causing any damage.

**Capillary (Dermal) Puncture Steps**

The process of collecting a sample via a capillary process is much different than that of a vein. When using this type of retrieval method, the order of draw differs. The use of this type of collection is common with children under the age of one, but it can also be used for people who have special conditions, or for blood testing that only requires a small amount of blood to be drawn from the site. By adhering to the steps listed below, the risk of injury and other complications can be avoided.

1.  Prior to starting the collection process, the technician should review the form provided by the physician.

2.  All of the materials needed for the testing process should be collected prior to starting the capillary testing process. This includes puncture device, gloves, mask, collection tubes, gauze, bandages, cleaning agents, and the other materials for the collection process from start to finish.

3.  Select the proper lancet for the collection. The lavender lancet has a 1.5 mm puncture tool, while the blue has a 2.0 mm one. The blue lancet is used when more than two drops of blood are needed for the collection process.

4. Place all tools on the tray. Along with the lancet, all the tools needed or the process of collecting the sample must be placed upon the tray prior to starting the process. The tray must include all materials used to complete the process of collecting the specimen, from the start of the process to the end. These include:

   - Gas tubes

   - Slides

   - EDTA

   - Heparin

   - Serum (red top or amber top with red serum)

5. Once the materials are collected, the patient identification process must be completed, as needed, with all of the testing procedures used. This includes:

   - Asking the patient's name

   - Checking the patients ID bracelet

   - Comparing results with the information on the order form provided by the physician

6. Select the proper capillary area. The most common area of withdrawal is the hand, and the finger of the hand should meet the specifications set forth within the safety rules. For infants, the heel may be used for the draw, but this area is seldom used for those above the age of one, unless there is severe scarring, burning, or other issues with the skin present on the third and fourth finger of the hand.

7. Prepare the finger (or heel) by cleaning it with the appropriate agent. Then grasp the finger and puncture it with the lancing device that is appropriate for the collection.

8. Once the puncture has been made, the first drop of blood must be wiped away, as this contains too much tissue, and then the collection device can be filled with the sample that is collected.

9. Once the blood is collected, properly seal the container in order to prevent contamination of the collected specimen or oxygen from coming in contact with the collected sample.

10. After the sample is collected, the patient must hold a piece of gauze on the puncture site. The gauze will be left with the patient while the specimens are labeled with the correct labels. Labeling the sample upon collection is required before completing any further steps.

11. After the labels have been applied to the samples, they can be placed in the appropriate areas, and then the materials used for the testing process must be disposed of properly.

12. Apply a bandage to the area where the gauze is present, by first checking to ensure that the area if not bleeding too much, and then applying the bandage over the area with a light pressure that will take over holding the bandage in place.

13. Dispose of the puncture device in the correct container upon completion of the collection. Also, dispose of any materials that were used during the test in order to stop the risk of infection, injury, or illness to all parties involved within the test collection process.

14. After the materials have been disposed of, the technician must return to the patient, remove the gauze and check the site. If the area has slowed down with bleeding, the gauze will be reapplied to the site, a bandage will be applied to keep the gauze in place for a period of at least 5 to 10 minutes.

15. Remove the gloves used for the testing, and then thoroughly wash your hands prior to moving to the next patient.

In some cases, special specimen requirements may be set in place. When this type of situation is present, there are certain steps that will need to be taken to ensure proper collection of the sample material.

**Capillary Collection Lancets**

When the collecting a capillary specimen from the heel, the order of collection remains the same, but the lancet size varies. The lancet used for taking a sample from the heel can be:

- 2.5MM (green) for full-term

- 1.75MM (purple) for neonatal

- 1.2MM (blue) for neonatal babies less than 1000g

## Candidates for Capillary Collection

While this process of testing is recommended for infants, it is also done for those who meet certain medical requirements. This type of testing method can be used on patients who fit within one or more of the following categories:

- Patients with veins that are difficult to access, fragile, or considered to be superficial.

- Patients who have had multiple attempts of drawing blood, but the draws were unsuccessful. For some, further venipuncture may be needed depending on the volume of blood that must be collected.

If only a small collection is needed, a capillary collection will be sufficient for patients who:

- Are extremely obese

- Have bruising or scarring present at the venipuncture site

- Have received IVs in both arms

- Need to have blood tests done on a frequent basis

- Have a risk associated with deep puncture of the veins

- Are getting a test that only requires a few drops of blood

- Are reserved for future testing, such as the need for an IV within the near future

## Circumstances when Capillary Collection is Inappropriate

Capillary blood collection is not appropriate for certain patients. This form of collection must always be avoided in patients who fit within one or more of the following categories:

- Patients who are currently experiencing severe dehydration

- Patients who have poor venal circulation

- Tests that require the use of plasma

- Testing procedures that require large volumes of blood

**Tests that Use Capillary Collection**

While capillary testing can be done for patients with certain conditions present, it is also a common form of testing for patients who needs particular tests performed. The following tests are generally done with capillary collection methods:

- Blood glucose monitoring
- Complete blood count testing
- Blood smears
- Neonatal screenings
- Neonatal gases
- Electrolyte testing

**Capillary Collection Sites**

Prior to performing capillary collection, the correct site must first be determined. While determining the area of collection for the patient, a few different things should be taken into consideration in order to ensure the best results. The amount of blood that is needed for the testing process is a crucial point of consideration. Additionally, the patient's age and the accessibility to the area where the blood will be taken should be considered.

When selecting the site for retrieval of the specimen, the area should be pink and warm to the touch. The area can also be warmed prior to the collection, but it should not have any of the following issues present on the site:

- Calluses on the skin
- Burns
- Cuts
- Scars
- Bruises
- Rashes
- Purple hue indicating lack of blood flow
- Swollen skin
- Infection

The most common area used for the collection is the third or fourth (ring) finger of the patient. The non-dominant hand should be used when possible, as the skin on this hand is generally softer to the touch and does not contain calluses. The second (pointer) and fifth (pinky) fingers should always be avoided when performing this test, as the skin in this area is too close to the bone, and damage to the bone within the finger can occur when the area is punctured with the blade like device used to create an area to allow the blood to flow out of the finger and into the collection device. The thumb should also be avoided, as this area of the hand has the presence of an artery, which could result in serious injury if punctured.

The heel is recommended for infants. However, when the test is being done on the heel, the bone within the heel of the testing site must be no closer than 2 cm from the area of the skin. When the bone is too close to the skin where the testing takes place, it can be punctured, resulting in damage. When puncturing the skin of the heel, the device should be inserted at a 90 degree angle, which will prevent contact with the bone, and also help to increase the amount of blood flow that occurs once the area is punctured.

When testing on an infant, the risk of injury increases greatly, and certain guidelines must be followed in order to prevent any injury from occurring. These methods must not be used with an infant in order to prevent injury or risk:

- The back of the heel

- The arch of the foot

- The fingers

- The earlobe area


When testing is done on one of these areas of the infant, it can result in damage to the bones, nerves, or tendons. For children above the age of one year, the guidelines change and testing can generally be done on the fingers, unless certain conditions are present, which make these areas risky for the child.

**Equipment for Primary Blood Collection**

The equipment necessary for the collection process must be assembled in a manner that meets the standard policy of the healthcare facility. The process of assembly must be followed in the order listed below.

1.  *Tray*: The tray used for the materials should be one that is lightweight, easy to move, and allows enough space on it for the various materials necessary to perform the testing process. According to the Standard Tray Policy for Phlebotomy Technicians, the tray used must meet all three of these requirements in order for it to be used.

2.  *Gloves*: There should be at least two pairs of the type of gloves used to test, in the event of contamination. Also, there should be an alternative to the latex gloves, in the event that the patient has an allergy to latex material.

3.  *Hubs*: The appropriate disposable hubs needed for the collection process must be placed on the tray. According to the guidelines set in place by OSHA, any hub that has a security feature must be disposed of within the proper container. If a hub is reused after activation, it can pose a health risk to the phlebotomy technician and patient. Along with the hubs, transfer tubes should also be collected for testing requiring the transmission of the specimen. While there are transfer needles that can be used, the use of these hubs is preferred.

4.  *Needles*: The needle of the correct gauge must be placed upon the tray used for the collection process. If the size of the needle is not determined, the available of different sized needles should be present on the tray. The smallest needle size is G.

5.  *Syringes*: The syringes placed upon the collection tray must be sterile at all times. This means they must be in their original packaging. Any syringes that are not within their original packaging must be removed, as they are no longer considered sterile.

6.  *Collection tubes*: The appropriate tubes needed for the collection of the specimen must be placed upon the tray prior to meeting with the patient. All tubes must contain the additives needed for collection.

7.  *Tourniquets*: A clean tourniquet must be placed on the tray, and it should not be used twice. These are single patient use only, and can only be used again

on the same patient. If the work is done within an outpatient facility, this must be disposed of upon completion of the specimen collection process.

8. *Cleaning agents*: Two forms of sterilizing pads must be placed on the tray. This includes an alcohol pad used to clean the collection site area, as well as an alternative, which is typically iodine, unless there is a seafood allergy present.

9. *Gauze*: A few pieces of sterile gauze must be placed upon the collection tray. In some cases, cotton balls can be used in place of gauze, and these should also be available during the collection procedure.

10. *Ice*: An ice pack for application to the patient's skin in the event of certain issues arising must be available.

11. *Warming agent*: A heated pad must be available on the tray to help create blood flow during the collection process in those whose blood circulation is restricted.

12. *Completion material*: Bandages and tape must be placed on the tray for use after the puncture occurs. There should be more than one bandage for situations where the first attempt towards collection was ineffective.

After the materials have been collected, they must be properly assembled. The assembly of all materials must be done in front of the patient so that they can see that all of the items are sterile.

### Using a Vacutainer Eclipse

While holding both colored shields on the device, twist to remove the white shield. The white shield covers the end that will be screwed into the holder. Once the shield is removed, it should then be screwed into the holder, and the safety shield must be rotated back and out of the area.

### Assembling a Syringe Draw

Open the package that contains the sterile syringe, and remove the item from the packaging. Then attach the needle of the correct gauge to the end of the syringe by using a twisting motion. When a transfer needle is used for the collection process, the needle cannot be handled by the technician during the assembly process.

Instead, stabilize the needle on the tray with the collection tube, and using this method, place the needle into the syringe.

### Using a Push Button

Open the butterfly push button device from its original packaging. After it has been removed, the butterfly container must be attached to the vacutainer. This is done by removing the luer cap on the device and using a screwing method to attach the two. Once they are attached, the clear plastic needle sheath must be remixed.

### Verifying Equipment Quality

In order to provide the patient with the highest level of care possible, all equipment must be of the highest quality. There are different parts of the equipment should be checked in order to ensure it meets these quality requirements, including:

- *Sterile*: All materials used during the collection process must be in their original packaging in order to be deemed sterile. If the packaging of the items is opened, or the items are removed from the packaging, they must be discarded and a new one must be used. In order to cut down on the cost of materials, all items should be opened after they are placed on the tray, and in front of the patient who is receiving the test.

- *Expiration date*: Each item used within the facility has an expiration date that must be checked prior to using the materials. Any material that has expired must be thrown out and cannot be used under any type of circumstances.

- *Manufacturer defects*: All products must be checked prior to using them. This will ensure that all defective products are thrown out, and not used for the collection process. An example of a defect due to a manufacturer error would be the blood being able to drip from a collection tube, resulting in damage to the specimen.

### Tubes

The tubes used for collecting the sample from a patient vary. There are tubes that do not contain any additives, and there are tubes that contain special additives designed to be used with special types of blood testing. When choosing the tube to use for a sample, you must ensure that the tube you choose contains the additives needed to properly collect the sample and provide accurate results once the sample is sent to the lab.

- *Gold Top Serum Separator Tube*: This type of testing tube contains a blot clot activator and serum blood separating agent.

- *Plastic Red-Top Tube*: This tube contains the blood clot activator, but does not contain the separating agent or any type of preservatives.

- *Glass Red-Top Tube*: This type of tube does not contain any clot activators, separators or preserving agents. It can be used for general collection, or for blood donations.

- *EDTA Pink-Top Tube*: This is the preferred tube for collecting blood donations, and contains the agent EDTA.

- *Light Green-Top Tube*: This type of tube contains two additives, which are lithium heparin and gel-separating. It can be used for blood plasma collection.

- *Dark Green-Top Tube*: This contains sodium heparin, which is used for the collection of blood plasma, when whole white blood cells need to be collected.

- *Grey-Top Tube*: There are two additives within this tube, which are potassium oxalate as an anticoagulant and sodium fluoride as a preservative. This testing tube is used for the collection of whole blood that must perverse the bloods glucose.

- *Lavender-Top Tubes*: The additive in this tube is EDTA, and it is the preferred tube for molecular tests.

Once the tube for collection is chosen, the proper method of mixing the components must be determined based upon the type of tube used. Some tubes will need to be placed in for processor upon collection, while others will need to be inverted a specific amount of times to mix the agent within the tube with the collected specimen.

**Inverting Evacuated Tubes with Additives after Collection**

When the tube used for the collection contains additives, the tube must be inverted a specific amount of times in order to complete the collection process correctly. This motion should be gentle, as vigorous inversion of the tube can ruin the collected sample. The amount of times the tube inversion must be done depends upon the type of tube.

- *Gold-Top Serum Separator Tube*: Upon collection, the tube will be inverted one time, and then it must sit for a period of 20-30 minutes. After this time has passed, the tube will need to be centrifuged for 10 minutes.

- *Red-Top Tube (Plastic and Glass)*: These contain no activators and will not need inversion.

- *Pink-Top Tube*: Once the blood is collected, inversion must be done immediately 8-10 times, which will ensure a proper mixing.

- *Light Green Top-Tubes*: Tube must invert 8-10 times upon collection.

- *Dark Green-Top Tubes:* Tube must invert 8-10 times upon collection.

- *Grey-Top Tube:* Tube must invert 8-10 times upon collection.

- *Lavender-Top Tube:* Tube must invert 8-10 times upon collection.

- *Light Blue-Top Tube:* Tube must invert 8-10 times upon collection.

- *Royal Blue-Top Tubes:* Tube must invert 8-10 times upon collection.

- *Yellow-Top Tube:* Tube must invert 8-10 times upon collection.

- *Pearl White-Top Tube:* Tube must invert 8-10 times upon collection.

- *Special Collection Tube:* The number of inverts is based upon the type of tube being used. Refer to the testing manual if further information on special collection inverting is needed.

Injury due to improper use of the needle during the testing process can be severe. This type of injury is called a needle stick injury, and approximately 600,000 to 800,000 of these injuries occur each year. When a needle stick injury occurs, it can take a toll on the physical and emotional well-being of both the patient, and the phlebotomist or other professional who is taking the sample.

In 2001, there was an act put in place to stop the risk of needle stick injuries. Proper insertion and removal techniques are one important aspect of eliminating the risk of this type of injury. Also, other important steps are involved, including wearing the proper protective clothing, using precaution when working with infectious patients, and using the right method of collection for different patients based on their unique condition.

The World Health Organization (WHO) has guidelines set in place that help to ensure the patient's safety throughout the collection process. The first steps of proper safety for the patient include the use of protective gear while performing the testing on the patient, while also taking the steps needed to perform proper hand washing techniques, and eliminating the possibility of contamination during the resting process.

**Hand Washing**

You must memorize and internalize the following list of elements that comprise proper hand washing in a medical setting:

- Clean the hands with antibacterial foam or gel prior to putting gloves on and after taking them off. If the gloves should come in contact with blood, the hands must be washed with hot water and special cleaning liquid in order to prevent the spread of infection.

- The hands must always be cleaned between instances of contact with patients.

- If your hands come in contact with any contaminated objects during the process of testing, wash your hands and replace your gloves with a clean pair.

- Hand washing must take place after handling any specimens collected during the testing.

- Anytime you are returning to the testing site from outside activities, hand washing must occur, even if contact with a patient is not taking place. This will help to prevent the spread of contamination between the items used within the testing facility.

*Proper Hand Washing Steps*

1. Remove all jewelry from the hands and arms prior to washing them.

2. Turn the water on and adjust it to a warm setting.

3. Apply soap to the hands and wash in a circular motion for 2 to 5 minutes.

4. Rinse the soap completely off of the hands after washing is complete.

5. Turn the water off at the site with the use of a paper towel.

## Steps for Using Alcohol Hand Cleanser

1. Ensure that there is no presence of contamination on the hands, such as dirt or blood.

2. Apply one tablespoon of cleaner to the hands, or use the amount recommended by the supplier.

3. Rub the hands in a vigorous manner, ensuring that all areas are properly covered with the solution.

4. Continue rubbing the solution around the hands until the agent has dried.

## Standard Precautions and WHO Safety Measures

In order to prevent the spread of infection to the patient during the testing process, there are standard precautions set in place that must be used with every patient.

- When gloves are donned, do not touch other items around the room, other than those that have been collected for the process of testing.

- Provide the patient with a gown if you anticipate skin-to-skin contact at any point in the collection process.

- Use a new tourniquet for each patient you are providing with care. You can reuse a tourniquet on the same patient - it can be left at the patient's bedside if further testing is needed. However, once the testing is completed, and the patient is leaving the testing site, the tourniquet should be removed and placed in the trash, and a new one must be used for the next patient.

When taking a blood sample from the patient, the least amount of blood needed for the testing process should always be used. When too much blood is taken during the testing process, the patient can experience negative effects, such as dizziness and fainting. All equipment used for the testing process must be checked regularly in order to ensure it is in the best condition possible for the patient. Also, all materials that are used during the collection process must be sterile.

The patient should be provided with information on the testing process. Along with information on the basic principles involving the testing, the patient must be given information on all possible issues that could occur with the testing process. Based on the patient's age and current medical status, these complications may vary, and providing a complete list will ensure that the patient know the steps to take before and after surgery to ensure safety.

**Venipuncture Safety Measures**

The standards put in place for properly identifying a patient prior to performing the testing process must be used in order to ensure the testing is completed for the right patient. Venipuncture safety measures include:

- Select the vein that is appropriate for the test. This is done by applying a tourniquet to the arm and gently pushing on the vein to ensure it is in good condition for the specimen retrieval.

- If the patient's vein cannot be located, the alternative method of specimen retrieval must be used.

- With both form of testing, the phlebotomy technician must complete the steps needed for proper collection when providing the patient with care.

- Identify any allergies the patient may have prior to having contact with the patient. If there are allergies present, taking the steps needed to use alternative methods will ensure that the patient is kept safe during the testing process.

- Clean the site where the test will be performed in order to reduce the risk of infection. Then allow the site to completely dry in order to eliminate the risk of further complications. The most important part of cleaning the testing site is to ensure that you do not come in contact with the site once the area has been cleaned and is ready for testing.

- Perform the collection process in the correct fashion in order to prevent injury to the patient. Generally, a 16 gauge needle will be used for retrieval of the blood. However, the appropriate size of the needle may vary based on different factors related to the patient's case.

- Closely monitor the patient during and after the collection process. Some things to pay attention to while taking blood from the patient include a faint expression on the face, a pale coloring of the face, and any physical cues that the patient may provide to you. When a situation occurs that indicates the patient may have an incident occur, such as fainting, remove the needle and treat the patient in a medically necessary manner.

- After the retrieval process has been completed, the patient should be asked to sit in the chair for a few minutes in order to prevent issues due to rising after the retrieval of the specimen.

- The site where the blood was taken should be inspected in order to ensure the loss of blood has slowed down, and the process of clotting has begun.

- When the patient stands to leave the room, ensure that they do not feel dizzy or need help walking from the testing site in order to prevent injury to the patient after the testing process is complete.

- When drawing blood from a patient, you need to be aware and ready to face any complications that can occur during the process of retrieval.

**Capillary Collection for Newborn Screening**

When the capillary collection is taking place for a newborn screening, a special piece of collection paper is used during the process. This paper is called a filter collection paper, and it collects the blood sample by allowing the paper to come in contact with a single drop of blood. When the blood comes in contact with the paper, the paper will fill with blood, and it can then be used for testing. When doing this type of collection process, the most important part of the test is ensuring that the paper does not come in direct contact with the infant's heel.

## Bilirubin Capillary Collection

When collecting a sample for a bilirubin test, the blood collected cannot come in contact with light at any point during the testing process. If the infant is in an incubator, you should turn off the lights prior to preforming the test. Also, a special UV filter tube must be used to protect the blood from exposure to light during the process of collection. Once the blood is collected from the infant, it must be stored within a special container that protects it from any type of exposure.

## First Aid

All employees working within a medical facility or laboratory should receive the training and equipment needed to provide first aid to patients when necessary. By having the education needed to properly provide first aid to the patient, healthcare workers do not have to rely on outside sources. The first aid requirements that must be met at every laboratory include:

- A first aid box that contains the materials needed to provide assistance

- A valid first aid certification

- A copy of an inspection card

The first aid station present in the facility must be readily available to the technician. This means the station must be nearby, and set up properly in order to provide the right first aid care to the patient. The items found within the first aid box must be in good condition and inspected on a regular basis. Also, the box must contain the appropriate amount of materials, as specified by the board. When the materials within the box are used, new items should replace them.

In case of injury, a form must be present within the work area, as this is used for reference by the technician in the event of patient or healthcare worker injury. Other than the regular contents for the first aid box, the box should also contain gloves of varying sizes to be used when providing first aid treatment. Medication should not be kept in the box where the first aid materials are stored. Finally, the box of materials should also contain a cardiopulmonary resuscitation (CPR) mask.

When providing first aid to the patient, the injured area must be examined in order to determine the best method of treatment. The materials needed for the treatment can be obtained from the box, so treatment then can be given to the patient. In certain cases, such as the need for stiches, bleeding must be treated, and then the technician should call for assistance per facility protocol.

**CPR**

Many healthcare facilities and laboratories recommend that all phlebotomy technicians have an up-to-date certification in CPR in order to practice within the field. The CPR will need to be obtained prior to employment, and then it must be renewed every two years in order to ensure it is valid. When a patient is in need of CPR, the mask that is available in the first aid kit must be obtained and the application of CPR must start immediately.

CPR is used for a patient when breathing or heartbeat has stopped. By using CPR within the right time frame, the patient can be stabilized while waiting for the emergency crew to arrive to transport the patient to the emergency medical facility. The start of CPR must take place as soon as a problem arises, as avoidance of this process can lead to patient death and serious liability for the technician. The use of CPR is not common, but all healthcare personnel should be prepared in the event that this need arises.

When CPR certification is granted, the certificate must be placed in a location that makes it viable to the patient and other healthcare workers. When providing CPR to a patient, the use of the mask that is available within the first aid box must always be applied. This mask will ensure that both the healthcare worker and the patient are protected during the CPR process, as it works to create an effective barrier between the two when providing the patient will oxygen.


*C-A-B*

The process of CPR requires the proper use of steps C-A-B:

- Circulation (C): The presence of proper circulation within the patient is an important part of the CPR process. This involves learning how to properly place the patient so that circulation is not affected during CPR. Circulation is achieved through chest compressions.

- Airway (A): The patient's airway must be patent (clear) for proper breathing and administration of oxygen. Clearing of the airway is done through the proper lifting of the patients chin, placing the head in a manner that allows for proper air flow, and then placing the CPR mask on the patient so he or she can receive the oxygen during the CPR process. The patient should then be checked to see if normal breathing is present. If normal breathing is not detected within the patient, you can move onto step b of the CPR process.

- Breathing (B): In order to properly stabilize the patient through the process of CPR, you need to breath for the patient. This is done by forcing the contents of your lungs into the patient's lungs through the mask. The breathing process for the patient must be done in the manner taught during the training process. First, you must give the patient two rescue breaths, which are needed in order to see if the chest rises in the patient. If the chest does not rise after the rescue breaths are provided, the patient must be given another set of chest compressions, followed by two more rescue breaths. In between cycles, the patient's breathing and heartbeat should be assessed.

Once the patient is stabilized through the application of CPR, you can then call for help within the building if someone hasn't already arrived to the station. Once another person is present to look after the patient, and the patient is stabilized, the call to the right emergency professionals can be made. If someone arrives prior to the patient become stabilized, they should be instructed to call for help while you continue with the CPR process.

While collecting a blood sample from the patient, there are certain complications that can arise. When these complications arise, it is important that they are recognized right away in order to address the issue that is present, and take the steps needed to provide the patient with the proper care required for the complication.

### Hematoma

A hematoma occurs when the blood from the vein is able to leak from the area of penetration and into the tissue surrounding the vein. You can recognize this condition by spotting an apparent dark spot present at the area where the blood is being drawn from. When this issue occurs, it is important that the tourniquet is immediately removed from the arm, the needle is removed from the skin, and direct pressure is applied to the skin. After applying the pressure to the site for a period of two minutes, the area must be checked to ensure the bleeding has stopped, and then an incident form must be filled out prior to attempting to collect the blood from the patient for a second time.

To prevent hematoma, be sure to puncture only the uppermost part of the patient's vein. The needle must fully penetrate the area where it is inserted within the uppermost wall, which will prevent blood from leaking from the site of penetration and into the area surrounding it, such as into the tissue located around the vein.

### Hemolysis

Do not draw the blood from a hematoma during the withdrawal process. If the syringe has a plunger-like piece attached to it, do not force the plunger back too quickly when drawing the blood from the area of penetration. Avoid probing the vein during the collection process, and ensure that the area is completely dry prior to injecting the needle into the patient.

### Hemoconcentration

The presence of concentrated blood cells can occur while taking blood from the body, which can have a negative effect on the testing results. When hemoconcentration occurs, the concentrated molecules can cause a test to have a negative effect on the level of proteins, magnesium, ammonia, LDH, and some other products found within the blood.

To prevent hemoconcentration, avoid allowing a tourniquet to stay on a patient's arm for a long period. Additionally, avoid squeezing, probing, or massaging the area during the retrieval of the blood specimen. These actions can result in a concentration of larger or connected elements within the blood sample collected, which has a negative impact on the results once the blood is sent to the lab for processing.

**Injury**

An injury can occur to the nerve, muscle, and/or tendon located in the area where penetration takes place if the needle is probed or inserted into the area without the proper angle of application. Avoid these actions to prevent injury.

**Falls and Fainting**

There are two common causes of fainting during the collection of a blood sample. Some patients may become dizzy due to fasting prior to having the test done, and the fainting can occur shortly upon starting the retrieval of blood. Some patients will experience fainting due to the sight of blood.

The first preparatory step for this type of situation is asking the patient if they have a tendency to faint. If the answer to this question is yes, asking the patient to lie down during the testing process can help to eliminate an injury during the blood draw. While in the process of taking blood from the patient, there are additional steps that can be taken in the event of the patient fainting. These include:

- If the patient states he or she feels faint, or looks as if they may faint while you are drawing blood from the patient, you must take the needle out of the site right away.

- Ask the patient to lower their head and begin taking deep breaths. This can stop the patient from fainting.

- If the patient does faint, call for help and get the patient moved to the proper location.

- Applying a cold towel to the back of the patient's neck can help them wake after they have fainted.

- Offer the patient a drink such as juice for a quicker recovery, especially if fainting occurs due to fasting.

- When the patient wakes up from the fainting spell, an incident report must be completed.

- After a patient recovers from a fainting spell, determine if a second attempt of specimen retrieval should be performed on the patient.

## Infection

By following the proper standards set in place regarding cleaning of the venipuncture area, self-cleaning methods, and proper use of materials, the risk of infection will be greatly decreased.

## Lack of Blood Flow

When blood is not flowing freely through the area during the collection process, there are different steps that can be taken to improve the amount of blood flow in the area. The steps taken to increase the blood flow are based upon the type of testing method that is being used.

Venipuncture blood flow can be improved by repositioning the needle while it is present under the skin. This is done by moving the needle in a higher location, a lower locating, or ensuring that the needle is properly positioned against the vein wall once it is inserted into the testing site. If blood flow is still restricted, the tourniquet should be removed from the arm to see if this improves the issue. However, if the issue is still present, a new location for retrieval of the specimen should be determined by the technician.

With a capillary collection, the blood flow can be significantly decreased. When this occurs, you can warm the area where the blood is being drawn in order to improve the flow by up to seven times. The warming of the area can be done with a warm cloth, or a warming pad, applied to the area for under a minute prior to using the disposal puncture device to retrieve the specimen.

## Inability to Collect Sample

There are different reasons why the blood may not be collecting properly within the tube. If the lack of proper collection is not due to lack of blood flow, there may be an issue with the tube used for collecting the sample. For tubes that use vacuum suction to collect the specimen, the vacuum feature may be damaged within the tube, and it may not work properly to collect the blood. In this type of situation, removing the tube from the syringe and replacing it with a new tube can fix the issue. By having extra tubes close by during the process of collection, changing the tube in this type of situation can be done rather easily.

Another common reason for lack of proper collection is due to improper insertion of the needle. If you suspect that the needle is not properly inserted into the site, removing the needle from the area and re-injecting it into the site should correct the issue and get the blood flowing in the area. It is important that you do not dig at the vein in order to collect the blood when the collection is not working, as this can damage nerves, tissues, and tendons.

## Identifying Petechiae

Prior to taking blood from the patient, the skin must be examined in order to rule out the presence of petechiae. If the skin where the blood is being drawn from has small red dots on it, then the skin in the area may have broken blood vessels present under it, which can result in this condition. Petechiae occur as a result of coagulation issues with the skin, or due to abnormalities within the body.

When an area of the skin with petechiae is used for testing, the patient may have excessive bleeding occur, which could result in serious complications for the patient. By being aware of this issue prior to taking blood from the site, the technician will be able to prepare for this situation and take the steps needed to prevent excessive blood loss. When this issue is present, the technician must ensure that blood loss has stopped prior to leaving the patient. If blood loss continues for a prolonged period of time, the technician must call a medical professional in order to address the condition.

## Nerve Damage

The patient may experience a sharp, pinching feeling in the area where the needle is inserted. This can indicate the presence of nerve damage, and the needle needs to be removed from the site immediately in order to prevent the damage from getting worse. If this does occur, an incident report will need to be filed and the patient may need to have physical therapy in order to help the nerve within the area repair.

## Mastectomy

When a woman has had one or both breasts removed, she will need to have the lymph nodes in the body removed as well. When the lymph nodes are removed from the body, it can affect the rate of blood flow present in the arms. This can lead to accumulation of the tissue located within the arms, which can cause an infection to occur during the process of taking blood from the body.

This tissue is present within the body in a clear form, and when withdrawing blood from one of the arms, the liquid can be removed along with the blood, which can have a negative impact on the test results. When this condition is present, the patient may be able to designate another arm for the testing process. If both arms have this liquid present within the tissue, the testing process may need to be completed in the form of a finger prick.

## Obesity

In patients who are severely obese, the veins can be located deep within the arm area, and puncturing the vein may be very difficult. The technician may insert the needle based on the knowledge of anatomy, and may not come in contact with the vein. When this occurs, the blood will not be properly drawn from the area, and the risk of infection or injury is increased. In order to prevent these risks from occurring, the use of a finger prick device should be considered, especially if the vein is not visually available after applying the tourniquet to the area where the administration of the needle should take place.

## Collapsed Vein

When the plunger attached to the syringe is pulled back with too much force, the vein can collapse. When this occurs, the needle must be retracted from the vein, as a collapsed vein will restrict the blood from flowing through the vein, and the sample will not be able to flow from the vein and into the test tube. This can also be caused by using a vein that is too small for the testing process, and using a new vein for the sample collection can remedy the issue.

## Allergies

If a patient is allergic to one of the materials used for the testing, the proper medical treatment must be provided to the patient right away in order to prevent the risk of a severe allergic reaction. Some patients may have an allergy to the alcohol used to clean the area, while others can have an allergy to latex. By asking the patient if they have any allergies prior to performing the test, the testing process can be completed with a much lower risk of an allergic reaction. In the case of an allergy to the materials used in the testing process, the alternatives available should be used. This includes the use of non-latex gloves, and iodine solution used in place of the standard alcohol.

## Thrombosis

Thrombosis is present in the blood as a solid clot. When this condition occurs, drawing blood from the vein may be very difficult, even when the steps taken to improve the circulation of blood flow within the area. In this type of situation, the needle should be removed from the arm, and a new area of penetration should be determined. In some cases, this method of withdrawal will be impossible, and the patient will need to have the alternative form of drawing blood, such as a capillary collection.

## Infections

If there is the presence of an infection, the proper safety protocols for infectious patients must be practiced to the fullest degree. This includes wearing the correct protective gear needed to protect you from infection while drawing blood, which also includes a face mask due to the ability to contract an infection with airborne particles released into the air during the process of drawing blood from the patient. Special equipment may also be used to draw blood from the site and reduce the risk of infection.

## Basal State Anomalies

The basal state of the patient must be closely monitored during the process of testing. This is the patient's current health condition based on the state recorded 12 hours after having the last meal or upon waking in the morning. The basal state needs to be level in order to get the right results from the specimen collected from the patient, and to prevent patient risk. There are specific conditions that can affect the patient's basal state.

## Serum Identity

Serum collected from the patient is generally clear in color. However, when certain problems are present, serum can appear cloudy or milky in appearance. The following condition can affect the appearance of serum:

- Improper basal state

- Bacteria present in the specimen

- Fat within the specimen due to eating fatty foods

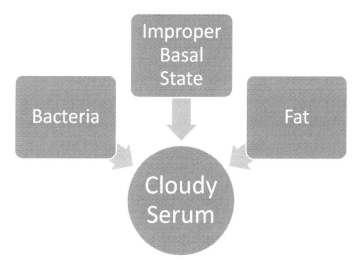

## Stress

If the patient is showing signs of stress, this can cause certain materials within the body to show higher than normal. This includes the presence of high levels of iron, abnormal adrenal hormones, glucose, insulin, and additional substances. If the patient's stress is higher than normal (due to anxiety about the procedure), the patient may need to learn certain relaxation methods in order to ensure the test produces correct results.

## Seizure

While rare, seizure can occur during the process of collecting blood. If a patient has a seizure, the needle must be removed immediately, and you must seek emergency medical attention immediately. It is important that nothing is near the patient's mouth in this situation, and that the patient be turned on their side in order to prevent chewing or choking on the tongue.

## Nausea

When nausea occurs, the patient can make a quick movement to vomit, which can cause injury to occur in the area where the needle is administer. In order to protect the patient, signs of nausea should be monitored. This includes a pale look in the face or the patient expressing that they are feeling queasy. The test should not be completed until the nausea has diminished.

For some specialized tests, the method of drawing the blood will differ from that normally used. By following the methods listed, the phlebotomy technician will avoid harm to the patient, improper testing results and legal issues.

**Preparing Peripheral Blood Smears**

Peripheral blood smears require a blood sample of 20 mm to be taken with the normal method of draw. Once the sample is collected, the blood is placed onto a slide, and then it is spread across the slide with a device that spreads out the plasma, without causing any damage to cellular components. Once the blood is collected and placed upon the slide, it must air dry prior to being tested.

**Performing Blood Culture Collections**

Blood cultures are used to detect bacteria in the blood. When this test is performed, the blood must be collected within a vial that doesn't contain any additives, and then the culture is placed in a cup that contains specialized materials, which allow the bacteria or fungus present in the blood to grow.

All healthcare personnel must work together in order to provide the patient with the best care possible. In some situations, you'll need to help another technician with the blood culture collection.

**Collecting Blood Samples for Newborn Metabolism Issues**

Newborns are often tested after delivery. Sometimes, the blood must be collected to perform a full metabolic screening.  The following samples must be obtained when testing for this issue:

- Complete blood count
- Arterial blood gases
- Electrolytes
- Blood glucose testing
- Plasma ammonia
- Blood serum testing

**Performing Phlebotomy for Blood Donations**

The WHO has standards that must be followed before and after the collection of blood from a donor. This blood is used for testing the patient health, so the blood must be evaluated for infection prior to donation. There are a few different ways that the patient can be tested for infection when donating blood.

- A questionnaire must be filled out by the patient. This questioner will ask a variety of questions based upon the donor's current health, and any issues they have with their health. Any diseases or risk of diseases will be noted.

- The skin should be checked for infection prior to taking the donation from the donor. The signs of infection vary, and even the smallest sign of infection, will be cause not to allow the donor to donate blood.

- A sample of the donor's blood must be taken prior to the donation process in order to test for infection and disease.

One common cause of an infection spreading is skin contamination at the collection site. To prevent contamination, a cleaning agent of 2% chlorhexidine gluconate and 70% isopropyl alcohol must be applied to the site, and then the area will need to dry for two minutes prior to taking the collection.

**Avoiding Iatrogenic Anemia by Calculating Volume Requirements**

During blood donation, taking too much blood from one patient can result in iatrogenic anemia. In order to prevent this problem from occurring, the patient's weight and height must be calculated with the amount of blood that is to be drawn. If the risk of anemia is present with the blood draw, there are steps that can be taken to help prevent the issue.

- Smaller amounts of blood can be taken for certain tests. Pediatric tubes can reduce the amount of blood loss by as much as 47%. Prior to testing, the minimum blood requirement for testing must be configured.

- Return any dead space blood loss to the patient.

- Eliminate standard orders for blood testing on patients who cannot have the amount of blood needed drawn at one period.

# Processing

## Processing Samples

After the specimen has been collected using the appropriate collection method, the sample must be processed. A certain set of guidelines have been put in place in order to ensure proper processing of the sample that is taken from the patient.

### Labeling all Specimens

In order to ensure the highest level of safety is provided to the patient, all specimens drawn from the patient must be labeled in the patient's presence. There are certain sample labeling elements you must know in order to process the specimen completely and accurately.

- The label must contain the patients first and last name.

- The patient's date of birth must be placed on the label.

- The date of the collection must be present on the label.

- The technician who took the specimen must put their initials on the label.

- The source of the collection must be placed on the label.

The process of labeling involves collecting these different pieces of information and creating the label prior to collecting the sample. Once the label is created, the information on the label must match with the patient's identity. By asking the patient to verify the information on the label, proper labeling of the sample can be assured. While the name and date of birth must be present on the label prior to taking the collection, the time of the draw and the initials of the technician can be placed on the label after the collection process is complete.

The label must be applied to the sample immediately after taking the sample from the patient and applying gauze to the arm with a firm pressure. Once the collection is made, the label must be placed on the sample in the presence of the patient. The label must be placed on the body of the tube, and should never be placed on the lid of the sample collection device.

**CLIA and CLIA-Waived Procedures**

The Clinical Laboratory Improvement Act (CLIA) was enacted in order to ensure sample quality. This act sets guidelines in place that apply to large independent laboratories. After the initial creation, the law was expanded in 1988 to the Clinical Laboratory Improvement Amendments, which made these standards necessary in all facilities that perform blood collection procedures. Through this act, the quality, reliability, accuracy, and timeliness of the patients sample being sent to the lab is mandated and monitored to assure that these standards are met by all medical professionals.

- *CLIA-waved testing*: According to the guidelines set forth by CLIA, those who are performing CLIA-waved tests need to apply for a certificate of waiver. Laboratories will have random inspections completed to ensure that they are only testing with waived testing methods. Labs that wish to have this certificate granted to them need to pay a bi-annual see of $150 upon requesting the certificate.

- *Full testing*: For labs that are non-waived, CLIA has regulations that require all labs to develop, monitor, and evaluate the effectiveness of the policies and procedures used within the facility. The lab must also be monitored to ensure problems that are identified with the process are corrected with the right changes to meet the standards.

- *Proficiency testing*: One method of testing for CLIA-waived labs is called proficiency testing, which makes it possible for all personnel working to be monitored to ensure guidelines and requirements. Through proficiency testing, all people collecting the samples are following the guidelines, and the testing requirements provide the most accurate results. The test is done on a rotation basis among the technicians, and through it, any problems present with each individual can be addressed. The problem detected allows the facility to offer independent education to the technician and corrects the action that is not meeting the guidelines.

- *Quality control testing*: By performing the quality control testing process, the facility ensures that it meets the standards required by the quality assurance plan and CLIA guidelines. Technicians can use an external quality control device if their lab is not outfitted with testing devices featuring built-in quality control detectors.

**Transporting Specimens and Handling Requirements**

Those who are able to transport the sample collected from the patient must be trained in transportation requirements in order to ensure he or she meets the proper packaging procedures. The requirements of transporting and handling a sample must always be kept in mind during the collection process, and the regulations must be met to the fullest degree at all times. The sample collection must be done in a manner that protects the handler, the environment, and the sample collected through handling, preparing, and transporting the sample. Preparation for transportation requires the following steps:

1. All of the samples collected must be placed within a primary container that is designed for the sample. This container will have at least two different patient identifying labels on it.

2. The container must be sealed upon placement to prevent the risk of it being affected by outside airborne agents.

3. The sample must then be placed into a second container that has a warning label. The label on the container must state that the contents contain biohazard material. The second container is used to ensure that the specimen does not leak, should the first container become damaged. The need for a biohazard label is only necessary for bags or containers that do not show the contents inside of the container. For clear secondary containers, the need for a biohazard label is not present.

4. All paperwork sent to the lab must also be placed within a container that protects it from contamination. The container used should be in bag form, and it must be attached to the specimen, but it cannot be placed within the same container as the specimen.

5. If the collected sample is kept within a refrigerator prior to transportation, the refrigerator must be labeled as containing hazardous materials. The appliance must also be kept in an area where there is restricted access.

6. For specimens that require a cold environment, a third container must also be used for transport. This container is climate controlled, and will keep the sample at the right temperature during the transportation process.

7. Upon successful preparation of the sample, it must then be sent to the lab. The amount of time between collection of the sample and arrival at the lab is based upon time standards related to the urgency of the test.

**Preparing Samples for Transportation to a Reference (outside) Laboratory**

Sample preparation for transportation to a reference or outside lab must be done diligently. The method of properly transporting the samples varies depending upon the type of sample taken. All samples taken must have the proper labels prior to starting the transportation process. Steps for preparing samples include:

1. The first step is to use the correct method of collection when taking the sample from the patient. The proper equipment must always be used when you are gathering a sample, in order for the sample to be properly prepared. Different containers have different materials, and using the wrong type for the testing can result in inaccurate preparation of the sample.

2. When the sample is being sent to an outside location, the presence of a warning label must be clearly evident. This is because the sample will be handled by those transporting it, and these persons need to be aware of the possible risk that comes along with the transportation.

3. The sterile technique must be used when preparing any sample for transportation. This includes taking the steps needed to use only materials that are sterile during the testing process, and choosing containers that are sterile for the transportation of the specimen.

4. Place the specimen in a third container whenever possible. This will ensure that leak does not occur during the transport of the specimen. Generally, the specimen should be prepared for transport upon taking it, and then sent over to the lab for analysis immediately.

5. Ensure that all materials used for the collection and transportation of the sample are up-to-date, meaning that the expiration date found on the packaging hasn't expired.

6. Prepare the sample based upon specified conditions for proper testing. For example, if the sample must be kept cold during transportation, the third container used for the preparation of the sample should be a clean cooler unit.

7. Ensure items needed for the lab are assembled before transporting the container. The samples collected must have the testing slip, which will explain the types of tests required once the specimen arrives at the lab. All testing slips must be contained within a sterile bag that is attached to the sample.

**Explaining Non-Blood Specimen Collection Procedures to Patients**

When performing a collection that involves collecting a sample other than blood, the collection process must be fully explained to the patient beforehand. The different collections used include but are not limited to: stool, urine, semen, and sputum collection.

- *Urine collection*: The process of collecting a urine sample is done in two different ways. With either method of collection, the process must be explained to the patient, and then a sample cup provided.

- *Random urine collection*: This is done by collecting urine during midstream urination. After you collect the sample, the sample must be labeled with the same method of labeling used for blood collection samples (patient name, DOB, and patient identification number). The urine sample must then be placed within a secondary bag, which will be used to transport the sample to the lab. The testing form must be placed within the outer pocket present on the sample container. If the sample is not sent directly to the lab for testing, it must be kept within a refrigerated unit at a temperature of 28 degrees Celsius.

- *24-hour urine collection*: The proper preservative for the test must be collected and placed into the container. A warning that states the container contains hazardous material must be placed on the outside of the container used to collect the urine, and the additional container used for transporting the sample. With this testing process, the patient must first empty their bladder, and this urine must be thrown away. The time of the first urine must be recorded on the testing label. All urine that is voided within the next 24 hours must be saved within a container. Then, the final urine is taken at the end of the 24 hour period, and this is added to the sample that will be sent to the lab.

- *Stool collection*: The patient must be instructed not to take any form of antibiotics for 24 hours prior to the collection. The sample that is taken from the patient must be contained within a specialized clean container used for transportation purposes. The stools are generally collected within a two tube test, and each tube should be filled at least one day apart from the other. No more than two tubes should be used for the patient testing. When a stool sample is needed from a pediatric patient, a swab sample of the stool is taken.

- *Sputum collection*: When the patient is providing a sputum sample, the process of collection must be done by collecting a sample from the deepest area of the throat. In order to make this possible, the patient must be instructed to cough deeply and provide the specimen into the container used for transport. In cases where the patient is unable to complete the action, the use of saline solution or chest percussion must be provided in order to collect the sample. The patient must provide the sample first thing in the morning in order to yield proper results.

- *Throat culture*: The patient should be informed of the use of a tongue compressor and a stick swab for the testing process. The swap will use used to collect the sample from the posterior pharynx and tonsillar fossa. If there is any visible exudate present, the exudate must be collected with a separate swap and also sent with the culture. The patient should be instructed to avoid the use of antibiotics for 24 hours prior to the culture.

- *Semen collection*: The patient must be instructed to provide the sample into a collection condom or a container that is designed for the collection. The use of any additional materials, such as lotion or body oil, must be avoided, as these can have a negative effect on the sample and alter the results. Once the sample is collected, it must be sent to the lab within 30 to 40 minutes, and during transportation, the sample must be kept at room temperature.

**Handling Patient-Collected, Non-Blood Specimens**

Proper specimen handing and processing is a crucial step involved when the sample being used is a non-blood type and is taken by the patient, rather than the technician. The risk of contamination is much higher in this incidence, thus the directions for proper handling must be provided to the patient.

While these guidelines are set in place for all types of testing in order to ensure the proper processing and handling and accurate results, the patient must be informed of the proper handling measures. For example, if a urine sample is needed, the patient must be instructed on the proper way to take the test, such as a mid-stream urine where the patient starts the collection mid-way through the process of urinating. With all testing procedures, the patient must be instructed to wash their hands prior to collecting the sample, avoid touching the inside of the testing container, and place the container within the transportation bag upon collection. The criteria for handing non-blood specimens include:

- The container provided to the patient for collection must have a proper label on it. The label must have the information needed for proper labeling methods in order for the patient identification process to be accurate.

- The amount of the sample needed must be determined and discussed with the patient prior to sample collection. If there is a marker present on the collection device, the patient must be shown the marker and instructed to meet at least the minimum guidelines. For testing devices that have a maximum line, the line must also be shown to the patient in order to ensure the testing container is not overfilled.

- After the patient has collected the sample, and placed it within the transport bag, the lab technician must write the time of collection of the bag and also place their initials on it.

- After the sample has been provided from the patient, the proper storage and protection methods must be used prior to sending the sample to the lab. This includes, putting the sample in an area where it will be kept at the right temperature, and taking additional steps, such as avoiding light exposure. Any special requirements that must be met by the patient should be fully explained to ensure proper collection.

**Coordinating Communication between Non-Laboratory Personnel for Processing and Collection**

A high level of proper communication must be used when you are working with non-laboratory professionals, who will aid in the processing and collection of the sample. Good communication techniques are needed in all areas of the collection and processing of the sample. This eliminates improper samples, as well as safety and handling issues.

When a sample is received from a person who works outside of the laboratory, the sample will need to be inspected by a technician prior to being sent for testing. The lab must be called if there are any questions regarding the collection process, and then also when the sample has been taken. After the sample is inspected by the professional lab technician, that person will need to put their initials on the sample.

All safety hazards present must be clearly outlined through proper communication with other members of the staff. For example, any infections disease present in the patient must be brought to awareness among those working within the lab. If any questions arise, the technician should discuss these with the physician. The process of collecting the sample should not be completed until the questions are answered clearly.

For specialized samples, such as those taken for a crime scene investigation, communication must occur with those working to collect the evidence needed. Workers must be informed of any changes made within the lab, and provided with up-to-date information on the testing process. Due to the method used for testing in this type of situation, ongoing communication is necessary for testing that meets the set standards.

Most of the errors made with a blood specimen collection take place during the pre-analytical phase of the testing. While these errors can have some serious negative consequences, they can be avoided by taking certain steps prior to testing. These steps must be taken with all patients who are giving a blood sample, regardless of the type of test, atmosphere, or method of blood collection used.

1. *Patient Identification Error.* Identifying the patient prior to taking their blood is a crucial step. When you do not properly identify the patient, errors that can occur include taking the wrong type of sample, misdiagnoses of the patient's condition, and the need to take a new sample from the patient. To prevent this situation, the patient must be asked to properly identify themselves, as specified earlier in the patient identification process.

2. *Sample Dilution.* When drawing blood, the sample can sometimes accidentally be diluted by mixing sodium chloride (NaCl) solution with the blood. If this issue occurs, the results of the blood test will be altered and could result in both a negative bias to all parameters, and the bonding of electrolytes within the blood. This error can be avoided through the following steps:

   - Any sample taken from a catheter must be discarded three times the dead space prior to collecting the sample that will be sent to the lab.

   - Any blood gas sample that is taken should be drawn with the use of specified blood gas container, which has dry electrolytes within it.

   - If the sample taken has a coloring that looks like it may be diluted, the sample should be retaken from the patient in order to ensure accurate results.

3. *Venal Puncture.* While drawing blood from an artery, there is a risk of puncturing the vein in the area. When the vein is punctured, the blood will leak from the area, and even a small amount of venous blood mixed with the arterial sample will bias results. When the blood from the vein and artery mix together, the parameters are not suitable for testing. To prevent puncture of the vein while taking an arterial sample, the following methods can be used:

   - Use self-filling syringes to draw the sample. This type of syringe works to fill itself with the blood, but only when the sample is taken from the artery. If the vein is punctured, the syringe will not collect the sample.

- Use special needles, called short-beveled needles, which are much shorter than those used with a standard withdraw. By using this type of needle, you will be able to position the needle on the artery wall much easier, and the chance of puncturing a vein will be much lower. Use correct insertion method, which involves inserting the needle into the artery and using a 45-degree angle to ensure that the needle meets with the artery, rather than the vein.

4. *Air Bubbles.* If air bubbles are left in the sample, the oxygen can cause the sample to show inaccurate results when sent to the lab. Any sample that contains air is considered to be void. In order to prevent the presence of air bubbles in the specimen, the sample should be visually reviewed to see if there are any air bubbles present. If the bubbles are detected, or if they are present on the side of the testing tube, try gently tapping on the tube to dislodge the bubbles from the side of the tube and allow them to be removed. All bubbles found within the sample must be expelled right after taking it and prior to mixing additives with the sample.

5. *Blood Clotting.* The blood sample will clot together if the proper mixing method is not completed. If clotting does take place, the sample is not considered valid, as it will yield inaccurate results. To avoid the blood from clotting, use the sample device specified for that particular test, and be sure that devices that do not contain specialized additives. The dry form of heparin will ensure the blood does not clot, but if the liquid form is used for blood collection, it will dilute the sample and void results. To ensure that the sample is mixed properly with the heparin, the sample should be gently rolled between the hands after taking it at least two to three times.

6. *Hemolysis.* Hemolysis can occur when the sample is handled too roughly, or when it is cooled on ice. When either of the previous errors is made, the blood cells within the sample will rupture, and the electrolyte levels will be seriously altered. In order to prevent hemolysis the following steps can be used:

   - When the sample needs to be kept cold, avoid placing the sample directly on ice.

   - Use a gentle motion when mixing any sample.

- Avoid any turbulence to the sample by avoiding a narrow needle diameter, obstruction of the pathway used to collect the sample, and fast paced manual aspiration.

7. *Prolonged Storage.* When you take a blood sample, the cells within the sample stay active even after it is placed within the collection container. When the sample is tested after a prolonged period of time, it can show invalid results, and also those that do not currently pertain to the patients' health status. To avoid this issue, make sure the specimen gets to the lab in the specified time frame. The sample should be measured immediately upon collection, and for samples that need to be stored, conduct blood-age analysis, which shows the amount of time the sample has been stored. The sample should be analyzed within a time frame of 30 minutes. Any sample that cannot be checked during that time frame should be stored within a cool, icy area, but not touching the ice.

8. *Blood Separation.* Even when blood is mixed after the sample is taken, the blood must be mixed again prior to analyzing it. This is because blood that sits for even a short period of time will begin to break apart, and without mixing it, the sample will not be accurate. Prior to analyzing any sample:

- Mix the sample by rolling it in between the hands 2 to 3 times, and then inverting the sample at least one time.

- For samples that show separation visibly, the sample must be mixed 6 to 8 times prior to being analyzed.

- The use of metal ball tubes can ensure proper mixing of large samples prior to analyzing the contents, as the ball will move through the blood and mix it properly.

## Using Technology to Input and Retrieve Specimen Data

With the improvements made within the field of technology, the ability to input testing information and receive the results has advanced over the years. With a specialized piece of technology, the results of the blood test can be immediately provided to the physician, or other professional. This testing device assesses the specimen and records immediate results, rather than the original wait-time of 20 to 30 minutes.  This provides a number of benefits:

- *Increases department efficiency:* The machine provides real-time results, in the same manner as the lab, except at a much faster rate. This cuts down on the complexity of the testing process, provides results quicker, and decreases the amount of handoffs needed for collection and processing.

- *Meets established protocols*: By decreasing the amount of steps necessary, accuracy of testing results is greatly improved. The machine detects the most common types of testing methods used, records crucial values, and alerts staff when risks are seen, which improves the pace of proper patient care.

- *Improves patient care*: The amount of blood needed for these devices is much smaller than the standard collection amount. This can help to reduce the amount of blood loss to the patient, and also makes bedside testing an option for some patients. All data retrieved through the testing method is recorded for future access.

- *Reduces costs*: There are a few different ways cost is decreased through the use of point-of-care testing. The risk of an error is greatly reduced, resulting in less wasted material. Also, the process of transportation is eliminated, therefore transportation costs are eliminated. Finally, traditional testing methods can be eliminated, making the tests cheaper for the lab.

## Reporting Critical Values for Point-of-Care Testing

When point-of-care testing is used, and crucial values are detected, the results will be immediately sent over to the medical professionals responsible for the patient's well-being. The technology used for point-of-care testing can quickly detect life-threatening issues found in the blood sample, and the patient can be given immediate care.

Critical values are calculated by comparing the results of the test with other testing that is done in labs world-wide. In order for the sample to be considered critical, it must state that the condition detected poses an immediate threat to the patient's health. The areas tested for critical values during the testing process include:

- Magnesium

- Potassium

- Sodium

- Calcium

- Hemoglobin

- Glucose

- APTTD

- PT/INR

- WBC's

- Carbon dioxide

- Bilirubin

The levels can be easily tested for point-of-care testing because they are generally quite similar in both adult and pediatric patients. The level of critical care drops (meaning the critical value was not reported to the appropriate medical professionals) has improved since the creation of the American Society of Clinical Pathology (ASCP). This organization sets critical values, which must be reported when they are seen, and these values cannot be discarded without the approval of a physician.

**Distributing Laboratory Results to Ordering Providers**

Once the laboratory specimen is analyzed, the results must be reported to the right providers. The provider ordering the test is generally the patient's physician. However, the provider can also be a nurse practitioner or physician's assistant. In order to properly distribute the testing results to the provider, take these steps:

1. Identify the provider to ensure the results are sent to the right personnel.

2. The lab that has tested the sample must ensure the results of the sample are legal and correct, in order for the results to be sent to the provider.

3. Using the laboratory information system, the correct method of providing the results to the provider can be used. The results provided may need more than the original order form and test result form. The form of test result delivery can be found on the order form provided for testing.

4. Results must be sent to all designed persons. Some tests will only need to be sent to one location, while others may need to be given to various providers.

5. After the results have been sent to the correct providers, definitive confirmation of delivery is needed, and the confirmation of delivery of the results must be recorded.

**Adhering to Chain of Custody Guidelines**

The chain of custody form is completed by the phlebotomy technician, or any other person who comes in contact with the sample prior to receiving the results. This is done to ensure only accurate test results are provided during specialized testing, such as DUI testing for alcohol levels found within the blood.

Chain of custody guidelines ensure the technician's ability to properly trace and safeguard the sample taken from the start of the collection process to the provision of results. There are different steps that must be taken in order to properly meet the chain of custody guidelines, which are based upon the type of testing that is done. These include:

- *Collection of the sample*: During the sample collection, the patient must be properly identified prior to the collection process, a written consent must be signed by the patient, and the type of test performed must be recorded, such as drug screening or forensic analysis.

- *Written request form*: When the sample is taken from the patient, the written request for the sample must be attached to it at all times. The information that must be present on the chain of custody form during the collection process includes patient information, type of sample, name of the collector, time and date of the collection, and the location where the sample was taken.

- *Transferring sample*: When the sample is transferred from one person to another, the person who has the sample in possession must write the time and initials on the chain of custody form. This is done in order for the form to be considered valid.

**Invalid Specimens**

The sample taken from the patient will be considered invalid under the chain of custody guidelines if the following issues occur:

- The chain of custody form is not present with the sample upon completion.

- The red seal used to seal the specimen container is broken.

- The chain of custody form is not properly signed in the correct areas by both the technician and the patient who is providing the sample.

- The patient identification information provided does not match the information that is present on the chain of custody form.

- The red seal is not initialed by the person who gave the sample.

- A white testing label normally used for sealing is placed over the red seal that is used to keep the sample protected from tampering.

## Forensic Cases

When the sample is taken for a forensic case, failing to properly follow chain of custody guidelines can have serious consequences. Generally, the time the sample is taken is the only opportunity for testing, as samples are often taken from a deceased person, and their body is sent to the morgue after the test is done.

## Clinical Cases

Due to the need for accurate drug or alcohol levels found within the patients' blood, the blood or urine initially taken must be used for the testing process. If the sample is taken at a later date, the results of the test will be considered inaccurate. When deciding upon the method used for clinical case testing, a few different things must be considered:

- The level of alcohol or drugs present in the system can change quickly with blood concentration.

- The use of urine is often advised over other testing methods when used for drug or alcohol testing, because of its ability to present accurate results. This type of testing is non-invasive, allows for the proper amount of collection to be done, has a simple method of preparation and testing, and the concentration levels of drugs or alcohol are higher when taken from a urine sample.

- Tthere are some disadvantages that come along with urine testing, including the dilutability of urine, the possibility that a recently-taken drug has not made its way into the urine yet, and bacterial contamination.

- Other forms of testing used include saliva and hair. However, these are the least common of all four testing methods, and are typically only used upon specific request.

# Workplace Safety

Proper safety is vital for healthcare workers and patients within the facility. When the proper safety methods are not used, the risk of injury to both the patient and workers is greatly increased, as is the risk of legal action against the professionals. Most healthcare facilities and laboratories have certain standards that are designed to ensure the highest level of safety at all times.

## Regulations and Requirements

OSHA has several requirements to ensure safety for everyone present within the facility. These standards have a direct impact on the healthcare industry in the following areas:

- Blood borne pathogens

- Personal protective equipment

- Eye wash protection

- Standard respirator

- A log of injury or illness regarding the patients

- Bio-hazardous waste

The standards specify that all labs must follow the same guidelines in order to meet the standards of the Clinical Laboratory Improvement Methods (CLIM). These standards ensure that the workplace is a safe location for everyone involved. The CLIM also created standards for the testing process that ensure a safe working environment.

The main area of focus under the OSHA guidelines is proper hand washing techniques, which are used to stop the spread of infection or disease within the facility. Cleanliness can help protect the patients and lab workers, and a clean environment is important. The testing area must be regularly cleaned with the use of the appropriate chemicals, and no eating or drinking within the testing site is allowed.

All materials disposed of must be placed within a container that meets the OSHA guidelines. These containers need to be spill proof, puncture proof, sealable, and be of red coloring. The container must also be labeled to show that the contents within the container are hazardous. The personal protective equipment used by the technician works to protect them from exposure during the process of collecting a sample. Gowns are also used to protect patients during testing that involves direct contact with the skin.

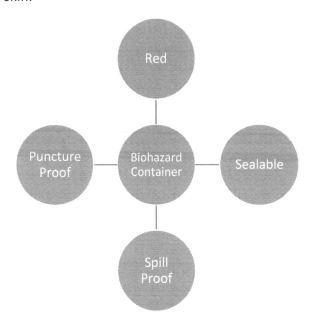

Blood disposal must be done in a manner that meets OSHA standards. All blood that is disposed of must be placed within the container labeled bio-hazard. If any blood should spill from the testing device, the area must be cleaned with a properly prepared bleach solution. Any containers for additional storage of blood, or other materials, must be properly cleaned and disinfected before they can be used again.

State safety guidelines must be met by each technician working within that state. While guidelines are generally universal, certain standards within the guidelines change based upon the state in which the lab practices. Regular review of the guidelines must be done by all technicians. Failure to follow the guidelines under this standard will result in serious consequences. Those who do not follow these standards could receive jail time and up to a $250,000 fine. Under these standards, if a technician sees another professional go against the rules or regulations, a report must be filed with OSHA, and then the proper method of investigation will determine the consequence of the determent from the guidelines.

## Adhering to Regulations Regarding Operational Standards

The Center for Disease Control and Prevention (CDC) works along with OSHA and The Joint Commission to create guidelines used to control the spread of infection within the facility. The CDC also has an up-to-date isolation procedure process to control the spread of infection. The Joint Commission has standards in place that focus on operations and patient satisfaction. These standards are comprised of four main areas which include:

- *Quality assurance*: Standards set in place to ensure the best care possible is given to patients who are being treated at the facility

- *Total Quality Management (TQM):* Designed to improve the satisfaction achieved by the patients by improving the services and communication provided to them

- *Quality Control (QC)*: Created to obtain accurate testing results from the sample collected by the patient

- *Risk Management (RM):* Contains a list of policies and procedures set in place to reduce health risks to both the patient and the technician

## HIPAA Regulations and Patient Privacy

Protected health information (PHI) standards ensure that patient privacy is safeguarded at all times. The Health Information Portability and Accountability Act (HIPAA) protects patients' privacy. By ensuring that the patient's privacy is met, there is no risk of discrimination against the patient, and the lab is protected from legal action or other consequences of exposing patient's private information. The privacy regulations under this law ensure that the patient's information is protected by following certain guidelines. These include:

- Anyone who is requesting information about the patient must properly identify themselves. If the person who is requesting the information is from a medical facility, his or her identity must be confirmed. If a person requesting information is not from a medical facility, his or her name must be on the HIPAA form filled out by the patient in order to receive any information regarding the patient in question.

- Any paperwork or electronic records that have identifying patient information must be protected with the appropriate methods. This includes putting the papers in secure location, blocking out electronic access to information in the computer, and ensuring that all paperwork involving the patients' health is only provided to those who are included within the immediate health care of the patient. The exception is when a consent form is provided by the patient prior to distribution of the information to the outside source.

- When using electronic devices for communication regarding a patient's care, the safety standards under the HIPAA regulations must be met. The HIPAA form provided by the patient must be kept up-to-date. Any changes within the policy must be discussed with the patient and then a new form will need to be signed in order to show that the patient had received the updated information regarding their patient privacy rights.

**Occupational Exposure**

The system for managing occupational exposure is designed to inform those working within a medical facility on the proper steps to stop the spread of an exposure and reduce the risk of injury. The exposure control plan used within a facility must always be up-to-date, and everyone working in the facility must be educated regarding these protocols. The following aspects fall under the occupation exposure guidelines:

- *Bodily fluids*: These include semen, vaginal fluid, cerebrospinal fluids, salvia, and any area of the body that is contaminated with blood. If the fluid from the body is unable to be identified, it is automatically considered hazardous.

- *Tissue or organs*: This includes those other than intact patient skin.

- *Any material that contains HIV cells*: If a patient has the HIV virus and exposure occurs, all fluids should be handled as if the they contain the virus.

- *Precaution*: The precaution used in the event of an exposure should be based upon the type of exposure. For example, the exposure must be determined to be airborne or a contact exposure.

- *Classification*: The exposure that occurs must be labeled with the correct level of risk present. Those working within the facility must also be classified according to individual risk. For example, those working directly with the patient are considered to be of the highest risk to exposure, while those who provide clerical duties are considered the lowest exposure risk.

**Following Transmission-Based Precautions**

In order to prevent an infection from spreading throughout the facility, both the possibility of transmission and the ability of obtaining the infection should be addressed. In order to cut down on the likelihood of the infection transmission, the patient must be met with the highest level of care when being tested. One small error in the testing process can cause an infection to spread from the patient or to the patient. Additionally, those working within the facility must create a strong immune system to fight off the risk of infection. They must have up-to-date immunizations, ensure good eating and sleep habits, and practice stress reduction techniques.

When a bio-hazard incident occurs within the laboratory, the phlebotomy technician must fill out the proper paperwork according to OSHA and the facility's standards. On the form, informational elements will include the type of incident, the details of the incident, and people involved in the incident. This form will be copied and kept on file by the laboratory supervisor.

**Types of Transmission**

- *Contact Transmission*: If contact is made with the exposed material, the proper method of precaution must be used. The area that made contact with the infectious material must be washed with a cleansing solution that meets the standards by OSHA.

- *Airborne Transmission*: For airborne infections or airborne exposure, those working within the facility must move to the designed isolation area.

- *Indirect Contact Transmission*: This type of exposure occurs when the infection is spread through an object within the testing facility. The area must be cleaned and covered, in the event of indirect contact exposure.

- *Droplet Transmission*: This occurs when a fluid from the patient is dropped from the collection site. If droplet exposure occurs, the area must be evacuated if the fluid is infectious. When droplet exposure occurs, and no known infection is present, a specialized solution must be applied to the area. Also, the fluid must be cleaned from the area in order for the space to be safe again.

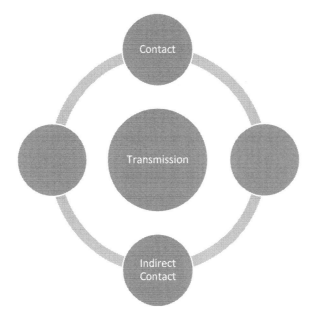

**Wearing Personal Protective Equipment while Following Standard Precautions**

Personal protective equipment is readily available to those working within the healthcare facility, and should be used at all times. This equipment is designed to protect the worker from infection while working with the patient. There are many different pieces of protective equipment used while working with a patient, and these pieces all work to provide different protective benefits.

A. *Gloves:* There are two reasons gloves are important protective gear in the laboratory setting. The gloves are worn to not only protect the patient while obtaining a sample, but to also protect the technician from exposure. The gloves worn by the technician provide a protective barrier when touching the different materials and body parts involved within the testing process. They also stop the spread of cross contamination during the use of different items. Lastly, the gloves protect the patient from transmission of infection when touching the patient and taking the sample from areas where open skin may be present.

B. *Protective facial equipment*: Facial equipment is designed to protect workers from infection material in the form of droplets or airborne matter. This equipment includes facial masks, goggles, and protective eyewear. The mask worn will protect the patient and/or phlebotomy technician from exposure to small drops of fluid, which can travel a great distance.

C. *Protective apparel*: This type of protective gear protects the clothing from exposure. It also protects the skin from exposure to the material that may present during testing, which includes body fluids and blood particles. The gowns used to protect the patient during the process of patient care may be disposable or non-disposable. They must either be disposed of upon completing of the collection process, or sent to laundry.

D. *Lab coats*: All technicians must be provided with a lab coat, which protects them during the collection process.

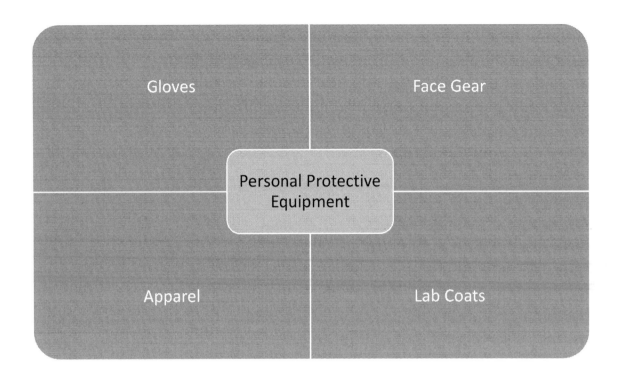

**Sanitizing Hands to Prevent the Spread of Infections**

The guidelines under the OSHA standards state that hand washing techniques are the most important process of infection prevention. There are two different methods of hand washing used when providing patient care, and they are designed to protect the phlebotomy technician and the patient. Hand washing must occur:

- Before and after each contact with a patient

- In between providing a single patient with different tests

- When the hands are contaminated with visual matter

- Before and after using the bathroom facility

- Prior to leaving the lab

- Before and after taking a break for lunch

- Before using the protective gloves and after they are removed

Washing can be done with the use of soap or a hand cleaner that doesn't require the use of water. When the hands come in contact with body fluid or blood, the use of water and a specialized cleaning agent must be applied. For cleaning in between testing, the alternative method of sanitizer can be used.

- *Water and soap*: When washing the hands with soap and water, the soap must meet OSHA's standards. The water must be turned to a warm setting, and then the hands should be placed under the water. After the hands are wet, the proper amount of soap as specified must be applied to the hands. The hands must be washed in a circular fashion, which ensures that all areas are covered during the washing process. After the cleaning is done for a period of two to five minutes, the hands must be rinsed with water and dried with a paper towel available within a closed container. The paper towel should be used to turn off the water.

- *Hand sanitizer*: The sanitizer used within a lab is of medical grade. The phlebotomy technician should use approximately one teaspoon of the sanitizer. After the product is applied to the hands, they must be moved in a fast, circulation motion, which will ensure proper dispensing of the product. The product must be allowed to fully dry prior to completing any further activities.

Hand washing with the proper technique is considered vital because the hands are commonly exposed to bacteria. When bacteria from an infectious person are left on the hands, the infection can spread from the hands and into the body through open wounds or nail beds. Also, touching another area of your body or the patient's body prior to removing the bacteria will cause spread and raise the risk of infection.

Safety standards create a safe environment for everyone within the healthcare or laboratory facility. By ensuring that everyone working within the facility has information on the current safety standards that must be used when providing patient care, the spread of infection and safety risks within the workplace can be reduced. The guidelines are forever expanding in order to ensure the highest level of safety care possible within all medical facilities.

## Practice Examination

**1. The patient must be greeted with a certain personal approach to gain a professional relationship with the phlebotomy technician, which includes:**

A. Dressing in a manner that portrays your appearance as well kept.

B. Maintaining good eye contact with the patient prior to starting the procedure.

C. Allowing the patient to have personal space and a comfortable level of contact prior to explaining the procedure.

D. Answering any questions.

E. All of the above.

Answer: E. All of the above.

Explanation: Choices A, B, C, and D all are important for a professional relationship.

**2. Why should the phlebotomist greet the patient, provide him or her with basic testing information, and answer all patient questions?**

A. This ensures that the patient feels well informed and completely comfortable.

B. This ensures that the phlebotomist is comfortable and confident.

C. This ensures that guidelines are met.

D. None of the above.

Answer: A. This ensures that the patient feels well-informed and completely comfortable.

Explanation: The phlebotomist should provide an introduction based upon the type of testing that will be done. This is accomplished by greeting the patient, providing them with basic information regarding the test, and then answering any questions they may have with the correct answers. This ensures that the patient feels well informed and completely comfortable by having all of their questions answered in the correct format.

### 3. How is laboratory testing information given to the patient?

A. Oral communication

B. Pamphlet

C. Handout

D. All of the above

Answer: D. All of the above

Explanation: The information provided to the patient is given through oral communication, or the patient can be provided with a pamphlet or handout, which gives information of the testing process and answers any additional questions.

### 4. Good communication with the patient is based on all of the following actions EXCEPT:

A. Eye contact

B. Good posture

C. Well-groomed appearance

D. Maintaining close contact

Answer: D. Maintaining close contact

Explanation: Good communication with the patient is based upon different actions, which include eye contact, good posture, well-groomed appearance, and respecting personal space.

**5. What Act states that taking certain information and communication steps will ensure the patient receives the highest quality of care possible?**

A. The Occupational Health and Safety Act (OSHA)

B. The Clinical Laboratory Information Amendments (CLIA)

C. The Patient Care Partnership Act (PCPA)

D. None of the above

Answer: C. The Patient Care Partnership Act (PCPA)

Explanation: Although not legally binding, the Patient Care Partnership Act states that taking certain information and communication steps will ensure the patient receives the highest quality of care possible.

**6. The "Duty of Care" standards ensure that the patient does not experience:**

A. Libel

B. Slander

C. Infringement

D. All of the above

Answer: D. All of the above

Explanation: The phlebotomy technician has a responsibility of meeting the "Duty of Care" rights of the patient before and during the testing process. According to these standards, the previous and following standards ensure that the patient does not experience infringement, slander, or libel, which can result in legal action.

**7. A patient is ordered to have a fasting lipid panel. What question should the phlebotomy technician ask?**

A. How old are you?

B. When did you last eat or drink?

C. Where do you live?

D. How much do you weigh?

Answer: B. When did you last eat or drink?

Explanation: It is important that the phlebotomy technician ensure the patient has met these specifications prior to performing the test. This means asking questions regarding the testing requirements, such as inquiring about the last time the patient had anything to eat or drink prior to the test. By ensuring the patient has met the testing requirements, the test can be completed, and the results of the test will be accurate.

**8. Of the following, which is an accurate example of "implied" consent for testing?**

A. The patient holds out his arm for a venipuncture.

B. The patient verbalizes consent for a urine specimen.

C. The patient signs a form for a stool sample test.

D. All of the above.

Answer: The patient holds out his arm for a venipuncture.

Explanation: Even if an informed consent form is signed, the patient must also provide a verbal consent prior to having the test done. If the patient refused to acknowledge the phlebotomy technician during the oral portion of the consent, then the technician cannot proceed. Implied consent is when the patient holds out his arm for a blood draw.

**9. The oral and written consent process should be completed by a legal guardian or parent if the patient is under the age of:**

A. 16

B. 17

C. 18

D. 21

Answer: C. 18

Explanation: If the patient is under the age of 18, the oral and written consent process must be completed by their legal guardian or parent.

**10. When a person states that he or she is the guardian or parent of a patient who having a blood test, what should the phlebotomy technician do?**

A. Assure that the legal guardian/parent is indeed serving in that role by obtaining a copy of an identification card and verifying this information by reviewing the medical record.

B. Assure that the legal guardian/parent is indeed serving in that role by obtaining a copy of an identification card.

C. Verifying this information by reviewing the medical record.

D. None of the above.

Answer: A. Assure that the legal guardian/parent is indeed serving in that role by obtaining a copy of an identification card and verifying this information by reviewing the medical record.

Explanation: Proof of identification must be obtained by the person who is providing the consent for the minor, and a copy of the identification card should be made and stored within the patient file. When receiving consent from a legal guardian of a minor patient, all medical history involving the patient must be reviewed with the caregiver in order to ensure the information that is on file is correct.

**11. Concerning phlebotomy, one of the main reasons why legal action is taken against a medical company is:**

A. Because proper consent was not received by the patient.

B. Because the needle was inserted too deeply.

C. Because the phlebotomy technician did not introduce themselves to the patient.

D. Because the wrong test was performed.

Answer: A. Because the proper consent was not received by the patient.

Explanation: One of the main reasons why legal action is taken against a medical company is because the proper consent was not received by the patient.

**12. JCAHO stands for:**

A. Joint Clinical Association of Healthcare Organizations

B. Joint Commission on Accreditation of Healthcare Organizations

C. Joint Corporation on Accreditation of Hospitals and Organizations

D. Joint Commission Association of Hospitals and Outpatients

Answer: B. Joint Commission on Accreditation of Healthcare Organizations

Explanation: JCAHO stands for Joint Commission on Accreditation of Healthcare Organizations.

**13. Hospital-based Patient Safety Goals of JCAHO should include:**

A. Verifying photo identification card

B. Matching patient I.D. bracelet with order form

C. Checking patient room number with I.D. tag

D. Receiving personal information via oral communication

E. Two of the above

Answer: E. Two of the above

Explanation: The Patient Safety Goals of JCAHO can vary based upon the location of testing, but should include two of the following: verifying photo identification card, matching patient I.D. bracelet with order form, checking patient room number with corresponding ID tag, and receiving personal information via oral communication, such as birthdate.

**14. What should the phlebotomy technician NOT do when identifying the patient?**

A. Call the patient "Sir" or "Ma'am."

B. Call the patient by his or her name.

C. Call the patient "Mr." or "Mrs."

D. All of the above.

Answer: B. Call the patient by his or her name.

Explanation: While properly identifying the patient, there are certain things that must be avoided in order to consider the information obtained proper and right. Do not call the patient by name.

**15. Where is the recommended venipuncture site?**

A. The antecubital vein

B. The brachial vein

C. The saphenous vein

D. All of the above

Answer: A. The antecubital vein

Explanation: The recommended site is the antecubital vein, near the bicep region.

**16. When performing a venipuncture, the phlebotomy technician should avoid all of the following EXCEPT:**

A. Area near the intravenous (IV) line

B. A scarred antecubital area

C. A swollen vein

D. An arm that was fractured in the past

Answer: D. An arm that was fractured in the past

Explanation: Areas to avoid include scarred, bruised, and/or swollen areas, those near an IV site, where previous blood sample testing was performed and not fully healed, the feet and ankles (unless otherwise directed due to certain special condition circumstances that can occur), and where a radical mastectomy is present, such as the left arm.

**17. The phlebotomy technician enters a patient's hospital room to obtain a finger stick blood sample. The patient seems agitated and confused. What should the technician do?**

A. Sit on the patient's arm to get the sample.

B. Restrain the patient's arm with a soft wrist restraint.

C. Seek help from another staff member.

D. Tell the patient he or she will be fine and attempt the finger stick.

Answer: C. Seek help from another staff member.

Explanation: If a patient seems agitated, confused, or hostile, it is important that help from another member on the staff be first obtained prior to testing in order to avoid injury.

**18. What structures in the arm resembles veins?**

A. Subcutaneous tissue

B. Tendons

C. Ligaments

D. Both B and C

E. A, B, and C

Answer: D. Both B and C

Explanation: Tendons and ligaments in the arm can be mistaken as veins. When checking the antecubital region, ask the patient to open and close his or her fist to avoid this mistake.

**19. Negative effects of testing can include all of the following EXCEPT:**

A. Fainting

B. Difficulty breathing

C. Convulsions

D. Striking out

Answer: Striking out

Explanation: The fear may cause the patient to experience several negative effects of testing. This can include fainting, breathing attacks, and convulsions. Striking out at the phlebotomist occurs when a patient is agitated or confused.

**20. In the U.S., how many deaths have been related to health issues that occurred from intense fear of needles?**

A. 2

B. 10

C. 23

D. 50

Answer: C. 23

Explanation: There have been 23 reported incidents of death related to health issues that occurred due to the intense fear of needles.

**21. Which blood collection method is least invasive and requires only a skin puncture?**

A. Venipuncture method

B. Dermal method

C. Phlebotomy method

D. None of the above

Answer: B. Dermal method

Explanation: The dermal method involves only one skin puncture, so the needle is not left in the skin long. This is used for infants, small children, the elderly, and other special circumstances.

**22. Which method of blood collection can take the longest?**

A. Dermal method for only a glucose test

B. Dermal method for multiple tests

C. Venipuncture method for only a glucose test

D. Venipuncture for multiple tests

Answer: B. Dermal method for multiple tests

Explanation: Due to the method of collection, the dermal method of testing takes longer to complete, and could actually pose a greater risk to people within a certain category.

**23. Which testing method requires the most blood?**

A. A dermal method for glucose

B. A venipuncture method for glucose

C. A phlebotomy method for glucose

D. None of the above

Answer: A. A dermal method for a glucose

Explanation: The amount of blood needed for a dermal testing method is less than that of a venipuncture.

**24. What can happen to blood during the dermal method collection process that would render a faulty result?**

A. Carbon dioxide meets with the blood and clots it.

B. Oxygen meets with the blood and clots it.

C. Rapid collection ruins the specimen.

D. All of the above.

Answer: B. Oxygen meets with the blood and clots it.

Explanation: The risk of oxygen meeting with the blood is greater during this type of collection process, and the delayed collection speed can result in clotting of the blood while it is being taken from the site, and also having the blood produce a faulty result when sent to the lab. The amount of blood needed with this test is much less than that required for a venipuncture test.

**25. Damage to what structure can result in significant pain for the patient?**

A. Tendon

B. Ligament

C. Nerve

D. Venule

Answer: C. Nerve

Explanation: Hitting a nerve within the area of puncture is one issue that can occur without the proper assessment. When this occurs, they are will be damaged permanently, and it can experience a significant amount of pain.

**26. What is the purpose of cleansing the venipuncture or collection site with an antiseptic agent?**

A. Eliminate the risk of bacteria entering the skin during the puncture.

B. Remove any bacteria from the skin

C. Both A and B

D. Neither A nor B

Answer: Both A and B

Explanation: In order to prevent infection from occurring during the collection of the blood specimen, the site must be properly cleaned with the right agents. The agents used for cleaning the skin are designed to remove any type of bacteria present on the skin, as well as eliminate the risk of the bacteria entering the skin during the puncture, which can cause an infection.

**27. What is the most common form of antiseptic used to cleanse the collection site when obtaining blood?**

A. Alcohol

B. Povidone

C. Iodine

D. Sodium chloride

Answer: A. Alcohol

Explanation: The most common form of antiseptic used is rubbing alcohol, which is applied to the site in a specialized manner. While alcohol is generally used to cleanse the area, some patients may have an allergy to this substance. A phlebotomist must make it routine to ask the patient if they are allergic to the cleansing agent used in order to prevent the risk of an allergic reaction.

**28. Before cleansing the skin with an antiseptic agent, such as alcohol, what should the phlebotomy technician ask the patient?**

A. Have you had your blood drawn before?

B. Are you allergic to alcohol?

C. Are you allergic to gauze?

D. Have you ever used alcohol before?

Answer: B. Are you allergic to alcohol?

Explanation: The phlebotomy technician should ask the patient if he or she is allergic to the antiseptic agent.

**29. The phlebotomy technician should cleanse the venipuncture site by using which type of motion:**

A. Rubbing from upper arm toward the hand.

B. Rubbing from hand toward the upper arm.

C. Rubbing in a circular motion.

D. Rubbing in a clockwise motion.

Answer: C. Rubbing in a circular motion.

Explanation: The phlebotomy technician should cleanse the site using a circular motion, either clockwise or counter-clockwise.

**30. When drawing blood, what size area should be cleansed with an antiseptic agent?**

A. 0.5 to 1.0 inches

B. 1.0 to 1.5 inches

C. 1.5 to 2.0 inches

D. 2.0 to 3.0 inches

Answer: D. 2.0 to 3.0 inches

Explanation: When cleansing the venipuncture site with an antiseptic agent, start from the direct location of entry when cleaning with the anapestic agent, and then work your way out for 2 to 3 inches around the testing site.

**31. What is the reason for cleansing the areas around the testing site?**

A. Bacteria can spread, decreasing the risk of infection.

B. Bacteria can spread, increasing the risk of infection.

C. The site can become contaminated during a sneeze.

D. The site is more likely to remain sterile for a long period of time.

Answer: B. Bacteria can spread, increasing the risk of infection.

Explanation: Be sure to completely clean all areas around the testing site with the solution, and do not only cleanse the testing site alone. Bacteria can spread quickly, and by only cleaning the area where insertion will take place, the risk of infection is great.

**32. Why should the cleansed venipuncture site be allowed to dry before the needle is inserted?**

A. The antiseptic agent can cause blood clotting.

B. The antiseptic agent can cause air bubbles.

C. The antiseptic agent can cause irritation.

D. All of the above.

Answer: C. The antiseptic agent can cause irritation.

Explanation: After the area has been completely cleansed with the cleaning agent, allow the area to air dry completely prior to inserting the needle and collecting the specimen. By inserting the needle before the area has completely dried, the chemical can enter the skin where the insertion takes place, and the agent can affect the blood and cause irritation to occur.

**33. Certain things may need to be done prior to specimen collection. Which of the following is NOT an example of this?**

A. Taking the patient's blood pressure.

B. Taking the patient's basal temperature.

C. Listing all of the patient's medications.

D. Taking a picture of the patient.

Answer: D. Taking a picture of the patient.

Explanation: Prior to collecting the specimen, some patients will need to have certain medical states checked. This can include taking the patients' blood pressure, getting the basal temperature, and listing all medications that the patient is currently taking prior to taking the specimen.

**34. The primary role of a phlebotomy technician is to:**

A. Collect the blood specimens in a manner that is safe for the patient.

B. Protect the individual drawing the blood.

C. Meets all phlebotomy requirements.

D. All of the above.

Answer: D. All of the above.

Explanation: The primary role of a phlebotomy technician is to collect the blood specimens in a manner that is safe for the patient, protects the individual drawing the blood, and also works to meet all of the requirements, while also performing the task in the most cost-efficient manner.

**35. Which is the first thing the phlebotomy technician should do prior to inserting the needle into the vein?**

A. Selection of the correct sized needle.

B. Selection of the testing site.

C. Selection of the correct range of motion of insertion.

D. Selection of the working device.

Answer: B. Selection of the testing site.

Explanation: Prior to inserting the needle used for collection, the testing site will be identified during the patient preparation process. Once the area of collection is identified, the correct sized needle and working device must be determined based upon the patient. Once the needle is identified, it must be attached to the tube that collects the specimen prior to inserting the needle into the patient's skin. When a plunger collection device is used, the plunger should first be moved in and out, which will ensure a proper range of motion prior to inserting the needle and starting the process of collection.

**36. The tourniquet should not be left on the arm for more than:**

A. 30 seconds at a time

B. 1 minute at a time

C. 2 minutes at a time

D. 3 minutes at a time

Answer: C. 2 minutes at a time

Explanation: The tourniquet will need to be applied to the arm prior to collecting the specimen. This is done by wrapping the band tight enough above the area of collection that is allows the vein to properly display, so the needle can be inserted into the area. The tourniquet should not remain on the arm for more than 2 minutes at a time.

**37. Step 3 of the venipuncture process involves using the hand to grasp the patient's arm and stretch the area of skin where insertion occurs. What finger should you use when completing this step?**

A. First finger (thumb)

B. Second finger

C. Third finger

D. Fourth finger

Answer: A. First finger (thumb)

Explanation: Using the hand, grasp the patients arm firmly, and then stretch the area of the skin where the insertion will take place. Be sure to use the thumb when completing this step, as this will ensure that the skin is not stretched too far, which can result in an injury to the skin where the needle is inserted.

**38. When performing a venipuncture, what angle should the phlebotomy technician use when inserting the needle through the skin into the vein?**

A. 5 to 15 degree angle

B. 15 to 30 degree angle

C. 20 to 40 degree angle

D. 40 to 50 degree angle

Answer: B. 15 to 30 degree angle.

Explanation: Once the skin is taut, insert the needle through the skin and into the lumen of the vein, at a 15 to 30 degree angle. Check to ensure that the blood is properly flowing from the vein within the arm, through the needle, and into the collection tube.

**39. What can the phlebotomy technician do if the blood is flowing at a slow rate from the vein?**

A. Reposition the needle so that it is up against the vein wall.

B. Reposition the needle forward or backward.

C. Reposition the needle so that it is almost out of the skin.

D. All of the above.

Answer: A. Reposition the needle so that it is up against the vein wall.

Explanation: Reposition the needle when it is inserted in the skin by moving the needle forward or backward in order to start the process of blood flow. If the blood is flowing at a slow rate, reposition the needle in a way that ensures it is up against the vein wall, and allowing the blood to flow through the area without restriction.

**40. Lack of blood flow into a tube during a draw can be caused by:**

A. A damaged tube

B. Lack of tourniquet restriction

C. Poor angle of needle insertion

D. All of the above

Answer: D. All of the above

Explanation: Lack of flow can occur from a damaged tube, inadequate tourniquet restriction, and a poor angle of needle insertion.

**41. If a lack of blood flow into the tube occurs during a blood draw, what should the phlebotomy technician do?**

A. Remove the tube and replace it with a new one.

B. Remove the needle and try another site.

C. Move the tourniquet higher.

D. Move the tourniquet lower.

Answer: A. Remove the tube and replace it with a new one.

Explanation: With step 3, you are to remove the tourniquet from the arm if blood flow is still restricted after completing the previous steps, as this may allow the blood to begin flowing by stopping the restriction that was caused by the tourniquet. With step four and when using a vacuum tube for collection, try removing the tube and replacing the tube with a new one if no flow is present. The tube that is being used may be damaged, resulting in lack of flow, thus replacing the tube can stop the issue and get the blood flowing from the testing site and into the collection tube.

**42. After the blood is collected into the tubes during a venipuncture, what should the phlebotomy technician do first?**

A. The tourniquet should be removed.

B. The tubes should be laid on the table.

C. The needle should be removed.

D. Apply a gauze pad to the venipuncture site.

Answer: B. The tubes should be laid on the table.

Explanation: After the venipuncture specimen has been collected from the patient, lay the tubes to the side, leave the needle in the vein, and remove the tourniquet if it is still on the testing site. Then, apply a gauze pad to the area where the needle is inserted.

**43. While the patient is holding pressure on the testing site, and before labeling the collected specimens, what should the phlebotomy technician do?**

A. Ask the patient to hold gauze in place with pressure.

B. Dispose of the materials used during the collection process.

C. Place the tubes in a collection bag.

D. Label the collection bag with a biohazard tag.

Answer: B. Dispose of the materials used during the collection process.

Explanation: After the venipuncture, the patient should then be asked to hold the gauze in place with pressure on the testing site, while you take the steps needed to properly dispose of the materials used during the collection process. Once the materials have been disposed of properly, you must label all of the collected specimens with the appropriate label right away.

**44. OSHA is the abbreviation for:**

A. Occupational Systems for Health Associations

B. Occupational Safety and Health Administration

C. Organizational System for Health Administration

D. Organizational Safety and Health Association

Answer: B. Occupational Safety and Health Administration

Explanation: OSHA sets the standards to ensure that all individuals are protected from health risks during the testing process.

**45. To clean up blood spills and leaks, what cleaning solution is approved by the Environmental Protection Agency?**

A. Lysol

B. Citricide

C. Bleach

D. Ammonia

Answer: C. Bleach

Explanation: The Environmental Protection Agency (EPA) states that any material that leaks during the process should be cleaned from the area with a bleach solution or another cleaning solution that is approved.

**46. What ratio solution of bleach to water is used to clean up blood spills?**

A. 1:5

B. 1:10

C. 2:5

D. 2:10

Answer: B. 1:10

Explanation: The ration of bleach to water should be 1 part bleach to 10 parts water.

**47. How long should gauze be applied to the venipuncture site after the blood draw?**

A. 2 minutes

B. 2 to 4 minutes

C. 4 minutes

D. 5 to 10 minutes

Answer: D. 5 to 10 minutes

Explanation: The pressure applied by the gauze and the bandage will stop the bleeding quickly by allowing the blood to clot. The patient should be instructed to remove the gauze from the area of withdrawal 5 to 10 minutes after it was applied.

**48. To prevent hematoma, the phlebotomy technician should do all of the following EXCEPT:**

A. Puncture only the uppermost part of the vein.

B. Barely penetrate the area where the needle is inserted.

C. Fully penetrate the area where the needle is inserted.

D. Gently insert the needle into the patient's vein.

Answer: B. Barely penetrate the area where the needle is inserted.

Explanation: When inserting the needle into the patient's vein, be sure to puncture only the uppermost part of the vein in order to prevent this condition from occurring. The needle must fully penetrate the area where it is inserted within the uppermost wall, which will prevent the blood that is being collected from leaking from the site of penetration and into the area surrounding it, such as the tissue located around the vein.

**49. Which of the following can cause hemolysis during a venipuncture?**

A. Not drawing blood from a hematoma.

B. Forcing the syringe plunger back too quickly when drawing.

C. Not probing the vein during the collection process.

D. Easing the syringe plunger back when drawing blood.

Answer: B. Forcing the syringe plunger back too quickly when drawing.

Explanation: To prevent hemolysis, do not draw the blood from a hematoma during the withdrawal process. When the withdrawal is being done with a syringe that has a plunger-like piece attached to it, do not force the plunger back too quickly when drawing the blood from the area of penetration. Avoid probing the vein during the collection process, and ensure that the area is completely dry prior to injecting the needle into the patient.

**50. Which of the following is NOT a cause of hemoconcentration during a venipuncture?**

A. Massaging the tourniquet area.

B. Squeezing the tourniquet area.

C. Leaving the tourniquet on the arm too long.

D. Not leaving the tourniquet on the arm long enough.

Answer: D. Not leaving the tourniquet on the arm long enough.

Explanation: Hemoconcentration occurs from allowing the tourniquet to stay on the arm for a long period of time or squeezing, probing, or massaging the tourniquet area during the retrieval process.

**51. To prevent a patient fall, what measure should the phlebotomy technician take?**

A. Make sure the patient is standing during the testing process.

B. Make the patient stand up quickly following the blood draw.

C. Avoid letting the patient stand up immediately after the blood draw.

D. Ensure the patient has a drink of water before the process.

Answer: Avoid letting the patient stand up immediately after the blood draw.

Explanation: The patient can become dizzy or faint during the venipuncture process. By ensuring that the patient is sitting during the testing process, an injury to the patient can be prevented. Also, do not let the patient stand up immediately after blood is drawn.

**52. What is collected during a capillary collection?**

A. Interstitial fluid

B. Intracellular fluid

C. Red blood cells

D. All of the above

Explanation: D. All of the above

Explanation: The blood collected during the capillary collection method contains material from the patient arterioles, venues, and capillaries. It will also include blood cells, interstitial fluids, and intracellular fluids.

**53. What site should be used for a capillary collection when the child is 18 months of age?**

A. The heel

B. A finger

C. The antecubital area

D. Any of the above

Answer: B. A finger

Explanation: The capillary collection method is generally suggested when drawing blood from a newborn baby. When testing is done on a newborn, using the heel of the foot is recommended. The heel can be used until the child is of one year of age, then the process should be done on the patient's finger.

**54. Which of the following patients is NOT a candidate for a capillary blood collection?**

A. A newborn baby

B. An 88-year-old frail woman

C. A 44-year-old man who has had multiple venipuncture attempts.

D. A 55-year-old woman who has not had blood drawn in four years.

Answer: D. A 55 year old woman who has not had blood drawn in four years.

Explanation: This type of testing method can be used on patients with veins that are difficult to access, fragile, or considered to be superficial, as well as patients who have had multiple attempts of drawing blood, but the draws were unsuccessful.

**55. Which of the following patients should NOT have a capillary blood collection?**

A. A 27-year-old woman who has mild dehydration.

B. A 77-year-old man who has severe dehydration.

C. A 45-year-old woman who weighs 220 pounds and is 5' 5" in height.

D. A 48-year-old man who has a sore throat.

Answer: B. A 77 year old man who has severe dehydration.

Explanation: Avoid capillary collection with patients who currently experience severe dehydration, patients who have poor circulation within the veins, tests that require the use of plasma, and those testing procedures that require large volumes of blood to be obtained from the patient.

**56. Which of the following tests is NOT typically obtained via capillary collection?**

A. Lipid panel

B. Blood glucose

C. Newborn screening

D. Blood smears

Answer: A. Lipid panel

Explanation: Tests generally done with capillary collection methods include blood glucose monitoring, complete blood count testing, blood smears, neonatal screenings, neonatal gases, and electrolyte testing.

**57. Certain issues present on the capillary collection site can impede the collection process. Which of the following is NOT one of these issues?**

A. Callus

B. Scar

C. Freckle

D. Rash

Answer: C. Freckle

Explanation: The area can also be warmed prior to the collection, but it should not have calluses, burns, cuts, scars, bruises, rashes, a purple hue (indicating lack of blood flow), swollen skin, and infection.

**58. Why should the phlebotomy technician avoid using the second and fifth fingers when performing a capillary collection?**

A. There are more nerves in these fingers.

B. There are more tendons in these fingers.

C. The skin in these fingers is too close to the bone.

D. The skin in these fingers is too fragile.

Answer: C. The skin in these fingers is too close to the bone.

Explanation: The second (pointer) and fifth (pinky) fingers should always be avoided when performing this test, as the skin in this area is too close to the bone, and damage to the bone within the finger can occur when the area is punctured with the blade like device used to create an area to allow the blood to flow out of the finger and into the collection device. The thumb should also be avoided, as this area of the hand has the presence of an artery, which could result in serious injury if punctured.

**59. When puncturing the newborn's heel for capillary collection, the device should be inserted at:**

A. A 90-degree angle

B. A 75-degree angle

C. A 60-degree angle

D. A 45-degree angle

Answer: A 90-degree angle

Explanation: When puncturing the heel, the device should be inserted at a 90-degree angle, which will prevent contact with the bone, and also help to increase the amount of blood flow that occurs once the area is prepped.

**60. Hand washing must take place after:**

A. Handling the clean specimen collection materials.

B. Handling any specimens that are collected during the testing.

C. Putting the form in the collection bag.

D. All of the above.

Answer: B. Handling any specimens that are collected during the testing.

Explanation: Hand washing must take place after handling any specimens that are collected during the testing. Anytime you are returning to the testing site from outside activities, hand washing must occur, even if contact with a patient is not taking place.

**61. Proper hand washing should involve washing in a circular motion for:**

A. 30 to 60 seconds

B. 1 to 2 minutes

C. 2 to 5 minutes

D 10 minutes

Answer: C. 2 to 5 minutes

Explanation: For proper hand washing, the phlebotomy technician should apply soap to the hands and wash in a circular motion for 2 to 5 minutes.

**62. The most important part of cleaning the testing site is:**

A. Using a circular cleansing motion.

B. Do not come in contact with the site after cleaning.

C. Do not allow the cleaning agent to dry.

D. All of the above.

Answer: B. Do not come in contact with the site after cleaning.

Explanation: The phlebotomy technician must clean the site where the test will be performed in order to reduce the risk of infection, then allow the site to completely dry in order to eliminate the risk of further complications. The most important part of cleaning the testing site is to ensure that you do not come in contact with the site once the area has been cleaned and is ready for testing.

**63. Signs of fainting include all of the following EXCEPT:**

A. Paleness of the face

B. A report of dizziness

C. Faint expression on the face

D. Coughing and sneezing

Answer: D. Coughing and sneezing

Explanation: Because patients can faint during the collection process, the phlebotomy technician should closely monitor the patient during and after the collection process. Some things to pay attention to while taking blood from the patient include a faint expression on the face, a pale coloring of the face, and any physical cues that the patient may provide to you.

**64. Proper collection order for venipuncture is:**

A. Light blue top tube, lavender top tube, red top tube.

B. Blood cultures, green top tube, light grey top tube.

C. Additive tube, light blue top, lavender top tube.

D. Lavender top tube, blood cultures, light blue top.

Answer: B. Blood cultures, green top tube, light grey top tube.

Explanation: Proper order includes blood cultures, collation tube with a light blue top, additive tube with a red top, serum separator tube (SST) red and gold tops, sodium heparin with green top, lithium heparin with green top tube, EDTA with lavender top tube, ACDA or ACDB with light yellow top tube, and oxalate/fluoride with light gray top tube.

**65. Tubes that contain additive materials must be mixed by the technician via a light inversion, which should be completed:**

A. 1 to 2 times

B. 2 to 5 times

C. 5 to 10 times

D. 10 to 20 times

Answer: C. 5 to 10 times

Explanation: Tubes that contain additive materials must be mixed by the technician. The proper method of mixing the blood with the material inside is with a light inversion, which should be completed 5 to 10 times upon collection. If the tube is shook for a longer period of time, or the shaking is done in a vigorous manner, the specimen within the tube will be damaged.

**66. What type of paper is used for newborn screening?**

A. Tissue paper

B. Processing paper

C. Testing paper

D. Filter collection paper

Answer: D. Filter collection paper

Explanation: When the capillary collection is taking place for a newborn screening, a special piece of collection paper is used during the process. This paper is called a filter collection paper, and it collects the blood sample by allowing the paper to come in contact with a single drop of blood. When the blood comes in contact with the paper, the paper will fill with blood, and it can then be used for testing.

**67. What should be avoided when collecting a sample for a bilirubin test?**

A. Air

B. Alcohol

C. Light

D. Pressure

Answer: C. Light

Explanation: When collecting a sample for a bilirubin test, the blood collected cannot come in contact with light at any point during the testing process. If the infant is in an incubator, you should turn off the lights prior to preforming the test. In addition, a special UV filter tube must be used to protect the blood from exposure to light during the process of collection.

**68. If a patient faints during the blood collection process, what should the phlebotomy technician do first?**

A. Call for help.

B. Remove the tourniquet.

C. Remove the needle.

D. Lie the patient down.

Answer: A. Call for help.

Explanation: If the patient states he or she feel faint, or looks as if they may faint, while you are drawing blood from the patient, you must take the needle out of the site right away. If the patient does faint, calling for help and get the patient moved to the proper location.

**69. If the skin has small red dots on it, this is called:**

A. Hematoma

B. Petechiae

C. Rash

D. Hemolysis

Answer: B. Petechiae

Explanation: If the skin where the blood is being drawn from has small red dots on it, then the skin in the area may have broken blood vessels present under it, which can result in this condition. Petechiae occur as a result of coagulation issues with the skin, or due to abnormalities within the body.

**70. Why should the phlebotomy technician do when a woman has had a right mastectomy?**

A. Draw the blood in the right arm.

B. Draw the blood in the left arm.

C. Draw the blood from either foot.

D. Collect the specimen via the capillary method.

Answer: B. Draw the blood in the left arm.

Explanation: When a patient has undergone mastectomy on the right, the patient may be able to designate the left arm for the testing process. If both breasts were removed, both arms have excess fluid, so the testing process may need to be completed in the form of a finger prick.

**71. Hemoconcentration can affect all of the following EXCEPT:**

A. Red blood cell count

B. LDH

C. Magnesium

D. Ammonia

Answer: A. Red blood cell count

Explanation: When hemoconcentration occurs, the concentrated molecules can cause a test to have a negative effect on the level of proteins, magnesium, ammonia, LDH, and some other products found within the blood.

**72. During a blood collection test, common substances that patients are allergic to include all of the following EXCEPT:**

A. Latex gloves

B. Alcohol

C. Latex tourniquets

D. Sodium chloride

Answer: D. Sodium chloride

Explanation: Patients can be allergic to latex gloves and tourniquets, as well as cleansing agents like alcohol and iodine.

**73. Which of the following conditions can affect the color of serum?**

A. Stable basal state

B. Sterile specimen

C. Fat within the specimen

D. Glucose within the specimen

Answer: C. Fat within the specimen

Explanation: The serum that is collected from the patient is generally clear in color. However, when certain problems are present, the serum can appear cloudy or milky in appearance, such as improper basal state, bacteria present in the specimen, and fat within the specimen due to eating fatty foods.

**74. The supplies necessary for phlebotomy include both latex and non-latex gloves because:**

A. Some patients are allergic to latex.

B. Some technicians are allergic to latex.

C. Latex interferes with certain laboratory tests.

D. Latex gloves do not fit all people.

Answer: A. Some patients are allergic to latex.

Explanation: Because some patients are allergic to latex, the phlebotomy technician will need to have a non-latex alternative available.

**75. What does STAT testing mean?**

A. The collection should be done whenever convenient, and there is no rush.

B. The collection should be done as soon as you have time.

C. The specimen must be collected immediately.

D. None of the above.

Answer: C. The specimen must be collected immediately.

Explanation: STAT testing means the specimen must be collected right away. URGENT means the sample should be collected as soon as possible. STANDARD means the collection should be done in when possible, and there is no rush on this type of collection.

**76. If a large amount of blood is taken from a fasting patient, dizziness and fainting can occur. What can the phlebotomy technician do when this occurs?**

A. Offer the patient a warm towel.

B. Give the patient juice.

C. Allow the patient to lie down for 10 minutes.

D. All of the above.

Answer: B. Give the patient juice.

Explanation: For some patients who feel dizzy, providing them with a drink, such as juice, prior to having them leave the facility will help to increase their sugar count and prevent dizziness.

**77. Which lancet has a 1.5 mm puncture tool?**

A. Blue

B. Lavender

C. Purple

D. Green

Answer: B. Lavender

Explanation: The lavender lancet has a 1.5 mm puncture tool, the purple has a 1.75 mm tool, the blue has a 2.0 mm tool, and the green one has a 2.5 mm tool.

**78. The preferred tube for collecting blood donations is:**

A. Gold top serum separator tube

B. EDTA pink top tube

C. Glass red top tube

D. Plastic red top tube

Answer: B. EDTA pink top tube

Explanation: The gold top serum separator tube contains a blot clot activator and serum blood-separating agent. The plastic red top tube contains the blood clot activator, but does not contain the separating agent or any type of preservatives. The glass red top tube does not contain any clot activators, separators or preserving agents. It can be used for general collection, or during blood donations.

**79. What is the purpose of a warming agent or heat pack when drawing blood?**

A. To apply to the patient's skin in the event of trauma or injury.

B. To create blood flow during the collection process.

C. To decrease blood circulation.

D. To increase venous constriction.

Answer: B. To create blood flow during the collection process.

Explanation: An ice pack for application to the patient's skin in the event of certain issues arising must be available. A warming agent or heated pad must be available on the tray to help create blood flow during the collection process in those whose blood circulation is restricted.

**80. Which tube does not require inversion after phlebotomy?**

A. Gold top serum separator tube

B. Red top glass tube

C. Pink top tube

D. Light green top tube

Answer: B. Red top glass tube

Explanation: The gold top serum separator tube will be inverted one time, and then it must sit for a period of 20-30 minutes. The red top tube (plastic and glass contain no activators and will not need inversion. The pink top tube must be inverted immediately 8-10 times, which will ensure a proper mixing. The light green top tube must invent 8-10 times upon collection.

**81. Prior to using collection tubes and phlebotomy materials, what should be checked?**

A. The shipping date

B. The expiration date

C. The test date

D. The manufacturing date

Answer: B. The expiration date

Explanation: Each item used within the facility has an expiration date that must be checked prior to using the materials. For any material that has experienced, it must be thrown out and cannot be used under any type of circumstances.

**82. A peripheral blood smear requires what amount of blood to be drawn?**

A. 10 mm

B. 15 mm

C. 20 mm

D. 25 mm

Answer: C. 20 mm

Explanation: A peripheral blood smear requires a blood sample of 20 mm to be taken with the normal method of draw. Once the sample is collected, the blood is placed onto a slide, and then it is spread across the slide with a device that spreads out the plasma, without causing any damage to cellular components.

**83. How is a patient tested for infection prior to giving blood as a donor?**

A. Having the patient fill out a questionnaire.

B. Assessing the skin for signs of infection.

C. Testing the blood.

D. All of the above.

Answer: D. All of the above.

Explanation: The WHO standards must be followed before and after the collection of blood from a donor. The blood must be evaluated for infection prior to donation by using a questionnaire, assessing the skin for infection, and testing the blood.

**84. What type of anemia can occur when too much blood is drawn from the patient during a blood donation?**

A. Iron deficiency anemia

B. Aplastic anemia

C. Iatrogenic anemia

D. Pernicious anemia

Answer: C. Iatrogenic anemia

Explanation: During blood donation, taking too much blood from one patient can result in iatrogenic anemia.

**85. What measure can be taken to prevent iatrogenic anemia from occurring during phlebotomy?**

A. Smaller amounts of blood can be taken.

B. Dead space blood can be returned to the patient.

C. Pediatric tubes can be used.

D. All of the above.

Answer: D. All of the above.

Explanation: To prevent iatrogenic anemia, smaller amounts of blood can be taken for certain tests, pediatric tubes can reduce the amount of blood loss by 33 to 47 percent, and prior to testing, the minimum blood requirement for testing must be configured. In addition, the technician can return any dead space blood loss to the patient.

**86. What information is NOT present on the label of a laboratory specimen?**

A. The patient's first and last name.

B. The date the test was ordered.

C. The patient's date of birth.

D. The date of collection.

Answer: B. The date the test was ordered.

Explanation: The label must contain the patients first and last name, the patient's date of birth, the date of the collection, the source of the collection, and the technician's initials.

**87. CLIA is the abbreviation for:**

A. Clinical Laboratory Improvement Act

B. Clinical Laboratory Institution Association

C. Corporation License Improvement Act

D. Corporation License Initiative Association

Answer: A. Clinical Laboratory Improvement Act

Explanation: The Clinical Laboratory Improvement Act (CLIA) was put into place in order to ensure quality of all samples that are collected from patients. This act sets guidelines in place that apply to large independent laboratories.

88. With CLIA-waived testing, those performing tests should apply for a:

A. License from CLIA

B. Certificate of waiver

C. Both A and B

D. Neither A nor B

Answer: B. Certificate of waiver

Explanation: According to the guidelines set forth by CLIA, those who are performing CLIA-waved tests need to apply for a certificate of waiver. Laboratories will have random inspections completed to ensure that they are only testing with waived testing methods. Labs that wish to have this certificate granted to them need to pay a bi-annual fee of $150 upon request of the certificate.

**89. For full testing status, CLIA regulations require that all laboratories:**

A. Develop policies and procedures.

B. Monitor effectiveness of policies and procedures.

C. Evaluate effectiveness of policies and procedures.

D. All of the above.

Answer: D. All of the above.

Explanation: For full testing status, CLIA has regulations that require all labs to develop, monitor, and evaluate the effectiveness of the policies and procedures used within the facility.

**90. What type of laboratory testing involves monthly evaluation with a rotation of technicians?**

A. Full testing

B. CLIA-waived testing

C. Proficiency testing

D. Quality control testing

Answer: C. Proficiency testing

Explanation: Through proficiency testing, all people collecting the samples are following the guidelines, and the testing requirements provide the most accurate results. The test is done on a rotation basis among the technicians, and through it, any problems present with each individual can be addressed. The problem detected allows the facility to offer independent education to the technician and corrects the action that is not meeting the guidelines.

**91. When transporting laboratory specimens, all samples collected should be placed in a primary container that must be:**

A. Labeled

B. Sealed

C. Plastic

D. Both A and B

E. Both B and C

Answer: D. Both A and B

Explanation: All of the samples collected must be placed within the primary container that is designed for the sample. This container will have at least two different patient identifying labels on it, and it must be sealed upon placement to prevent the risk of it being affected from outside airborne agents.

**92. What type of container is used for specimens that require a cold environment for transport?**

A. A large container

B. A climate-controlled container

C. A red container

D. All of the above

Answer: B. A climate-controlled container

Explanation: For the specimens that require a cold environment, a third container must also be used for transport. This container is climate controlled, and will keep the sample at the right temperature during the transportation process.

**93. What type of urine collection involves a midstream urine sample?**

A. A 24-hour urine collection

B. A random urine collection

C. A drug urine screen

D. A urine cytology test

Answer: B. A random urine collection

Explanation: Random urine collection is done by collecting urine during midstream urination. 24-hour urine collection involves collecting urine over the course of 24 hours. A urine drug screen and urine cytology do not need to be collected from midstream urine.

**94. What should the patient avoid 24 hours prior to submitting a stool specimen?**

A. Red food dye

B. Aspirin

C. Naproxen

D. Antibiotics

Answer: D. Antibiotics

Explanation: The patient must be instructed not to take any form of antibiotics for 24 hours prior to the stool collection.

**95. When is the best time to collect a sputum specimen?**

A. First thing in the morning

B. Mid-day

C. Evening

D. Bedtime

Answer: A. First thing in the morning

Explanation:  The patient must provide the sputum sample first thing in the morning in order to yield proper results.

**96. What should the phlebotomy technician do when collecting a throat culture from a patient who has visible exudate present in the posterior pharynx?**

A. Swab the exudate only.

B. Swab the area without exudate, and collect a separate swab for the exudate.

C. Swab the area without the exudate only.

D. Swab both areas with one swab.

Answer: B. Swab the area without the exudate, and collect a separate swab for the exudate.

Explanation: If there is any visible exudate present, the exudate must be collected with a separate swap and also sent with the culture. The patient should be instructed to avoid the use of antibiotics for 24 hours prior to the culture.

**97. When obtaining a blood specimen, diluting the blood with sodium chloride from an IV can:**

A. Alter the test results.

B. Increase the test values.

C. Improve the test results.

D. None of the above.

Answer: A. Alter the test results.

Explanation: When drawing blood from a patient with an IV, the sample can be diluted by mixing sodium chloride (NaCl) solution with the blood. If this issue occurs, the results of the blood test will be altered and could result in both a negative bias to all parameters, and the bonding of electrolytes within the blood.

**98. To prevent puncture of the vein while taking an arterial sample, the phlebotomy technician can:**

A. Use self-filling syringes to draw the sample.

B. Used short-beveled needles.

C. Both A and B.

D. Neither A nor B.

Answer: C. Both A and B.

Explanation: To prevent puncture of the vein while taking an arterial sample, the technician can use self-filling syringes to draw the sample as well as use special needles, called short-beveled needles.

**99. To remove air bubbles from the testing tube, the phlebotomy technician should:**

A. Gently tap on the tube to dislodge the bubbles.

B. Shake the tube vigorously.

C. Mix additives with the sample.

D. Add air to the tube.

Answer: A. Gently tap on the tube to dislodge the bubbles.

Explanation: If air bubbles are detected, or if they are present on the side of the testing tube, gently tap on the tube to dislodge the bubbles from the side of the tube and allow them to be removed. All bubbles found within the sample must be expelled right after taking it and prior to mixing additives with the sample.

**100. What causes hemolysis of the blood specimen?**

A. Inappropriate collection technique.

B. Putting the specimen on ice immediately after drawing.

C. Not inverting the tube.

D. Air bubbles in the tube.

Answer: B. Putting the specimen on ice immediately after drawing.

Explanation: Hemolysis can occur when the sample is handled too roughly, or when it is put right on ice for cooling. When either of the previous errors is made, the blood cells within the sample will rupture, and the electrolyte levels will be seriously altered.

**101. Prior to analyzing a blood sample, the sample must be:**

A. Rolled between the hands 2 to 3 times.

B. Inverted at least one time.

C. Both A and B

D. Neither A nor B

Answer: C. Both A and B

Explanation: Prior to analyzing any blood sample, the technician should mix the sample by rolling it in between the hands two to three times, and then inverting the sample at least one time. For samples that show separation visibly, the sample must be mixed 6 to 8 times prior to being analyzed.

**102. Why is a chain of custody process important?**

A. It ensures accurate test results.

B. It ensures quality control.

C. It ensures professional collection.

D. It ensures proper reimbursement.

Answer: A. It ensures accurate test results.

Explanation: The chain of custody is form completed by the phlebotomy technician, or any other person who comes in contact with the sample prior to receiving the results. This is done to ensure only accurate test results are provided during specialized testing, such as DUI testing for alcohol levels found within the blood.

**103. The written request form of chain of custody includes all of the following EXCEPT:**

A. The patient's information

B. The type of sample

C. The reason for the test

D. The name of the collector

Answer: C. The reason for the test

Explanation: When the sample is taken from the patient, the written request for the sample must be attached to it at all times. The information that must be present on the chain of custody form during the collection process includes patient information, type of sample, name of the collector, time and date of the collection, and the location where the sample was taken.

**104. Of the following situations, which one would be an example of an invalid chain of custody specimen?**

A. The chain of custody form is present with the sample.

B. The red seal is intact.

C. The form is signed by the patient only.

D. The red seal is initialed by the patient.

Answer: C. The form is signed by the patient only.

Explanation: An invalid chain of custody specimen is one where the form is not present with the sample upon completion, the red seal used to seal the specimen container is broken, the form is not properly signed in the correct areas by both the technician and the patient who is providing the sample, the patient identification information provided does not match the information that is present on the chain of custody form, and the red seal is not initialed by the person who gave the sample.

**105. What should be evident on the laboratory sample when it is being sent to an outside laboratory?**

A. The technician's name and worksite.

B. A warning label.

C. The patient's name and date of birth.

D. All of the above.

Answer: B. A warning label.

Explanation: When the sample is being sent to an outside location, the presence of a warning label must be clearly evident. This is because the sample will be handled by those transporting it, and these persons need to be aware of the possible risk that comes along with the transportation.

**106. Which of the following can eliminate improper laboratory samples, as well as safety and handling issues?**

A. Good communication

B. Patient cooperation

C. Both A and B

D. Neither A nor B

Answer: A. Good communication

Explanation: Good communication techniques are needed in all areas of the collection and processing of the sample. This eliminates improper samples, as well as safety and handling issues. Patient cooperation is necessary for the testing process, but it will not eliminate safety and handling issues.

**107. Improved technology in testing devices can:**

A. Decrease the amount of handoffs needed for collection and processing.

B. Cut down on the complexity of the testing process.

C. Provide fast results.

D. All of the above.

Answer: D. All of the above.

Explanation: High-technology testing machines provide real-time results, in the same manner as the lab, except at a much faster rate. This cuts down on the complexity of the testing process, provides results quicker, and decreases the amount of handoffs needed for collection and processing.

**108. How has improved testing technology reduced costs to the patient and healthcare facility?**

A. The risk of error is increased.

B. The process of transportation is eliminated.

C. Traditional testing methods are readily available.

D. All of the above.

Answer: B. The process of transportation is eliminated.

Explanation: By using improved technology for testing, the costs within the lab can be decreased, because the risk of an error is greatly reduced, resulting in less wasted material. In addition, the process of transportation is eliminated, and thus so are its costs. Finally, the testing methods traditionally used can be eliminated, making the tests cheaper for the laboratory.

**109. How are critical laboratory values calculated?**

A. Based on WHO criteria.

B. By comparing the results worldwide.

C. By assessing life-threatening issues.

D. All of the above.

Answer: B. By comparing the results worldwide.

Explanation: Critical laboratory values are calculated by comparing the results of the test with other testing that is done in labs worldwide. In order for the sample to be considered critical, it must state that the condition detected poses an immediate threat to the patient's health.

**110. What organization establishes critical laboratory values?**

A. OSHA

B. CLIA

C. ASCP

D. WHO

Answer: C. ASCP

Explanation: The level of critical care drops (meaning the critical value was not reported to the appropriate medical professionals) has improved since the creation of the American Society of Clinical Pathology (ASCP). This organization establishes critical values, which must be reported when they are seen, and these values cannot be discarded without the approval of a physician.

**111. What risk is reduced when proper safety methods are used in the laboratory setting?**

A. The risk of legal action

B. The risk of injury to the patient

C. The risk of injury to the healthcare worker

D. All of the above

Answer: D. All of the above

Explanation: Proper safety is vital for healthcare workers and patients within the facility. When proper safety methods are not used, the risk of injury to both the patient and workers is greatly increased, as is the risk of legal action against the professionals.

**112. CLIM is the abbreviation for:**

A. Clinical Laboratory Institution Measures

B. Clinical Laboratory Improvement Methods

C. Certification of Laboratory Improvement Measures

D. Certification of Laboratory Institution Methods

Answer: B. Clinical Laboratory Improvement Methods

Explanation: The Clinical Laboratory Improvement Methods (CLIM) are standards that ensure the workplace is a safe location for everyone involved.

**113. Laboratory material should be disposed of in a container that:**

A. Meets WHO guidelines.

B. Is of white coloring.

C. Is puncture proof.

D. Is flexible.

Answer: C. Is puncture proof.

Explanation: All disposed laboratory materials must be placed within a container that meets OSHA guidelines. These containers need to be spill proof, puncture proof, sealable, and be of red coloring.

**114. Standards of The Joint Commission that ensure the best care possible is given to patients treated at the facility are called:**

A. Quality control

B. Total quality management

C. Risk management

D. Quality assurance

Answer: D. Quality assurance

Explanation: Quality assurance standards ensure the best care possible is given to patients who are being treated at the facility.

**115. Total quality management is:**

A. Designed to obtain accurate testing results from the sample collected by the patient.

B. Designed to improve the satisfaction achieved by the patients by improving the services and communication provided to them.

C. Designed to reduce health risks to both the patient and the technician.

D. All of the above.

Answer: B. Designed to improve the satisfaction achieved by the patients by improving the services and communication provided to them.

Explanation: Total Quality Management (TQM) is designed to improve the satisfaction achieved by the patients by improving the services and communication provided to them. Quality Control (QC) is created to obtain accurate testing results from the sample collected by the patient. Risk Management (RM) contains a list of policies and procedures set in place to reduce health risks to both the patient and the technician.

**116. The Health Information Portability and Accountability Act (HIPAA) protects:**

A. Patient's safety

B. Patient's dignity

C. Patient's privacy

D. Patient's health

Answer: C. Patient's privacy

Explanation: The Health Information Portability and Accountability Act (HIPAA) protects patients' privacy. By ensuring that the patient's privacy is met, there is less risk of discrimination to the patient, legal action, or other consequences when the patient's personal information is exposed.

**117. The system for occupation exposure is designed to inform those working within a medical facility on the proper steps:**

A. To stop the spread of an exposure.

B. To reduce the risk of injury.

C. Both A and B

D. Neither A nor B

Answer: C. Both A and B

Explanation: The system for managing occupation exposure is designed to inform those working within a medical facility on the proper steps to stop the spread of an exposure and reduce the risk of injury. The exposure control plan used within a facility must always be up-to-date, and everyone working within the facility must be educated regarding these protocols.

**118. Occupational exposure applies to all of the following body components EXCEPT:**

A. Semen

B. Cerebrospinal fluid

C. Saliva

D. Urine

Answer: D. Urine

Explanation: Bodily fluids that are considered hazardous include semen, vaginal fluid, cerebrospinal fluids, salvia, and any area of the body that is contaminated with blood. If the fluid from the body is unable to be identified, then all fluids are considered hazardous.

**119. What type of exposure occurs when the infection is spread through an object within the testing facility?**

A. Airborne

B. Indirect contact

C. Direct contact

D. Droplet

Answer: B. Indirect contact

Explanation: Contact exposure contact made with the exposed material, and the proper method of precaution must be used. The area that made contact with the infectious material must be washed using water that is warm to the touch, and the washing solution provided to meet the standards set in place by OSHA. For airborne infections, those working within the facility must leave move to the designed isolation area. Indirect contact is a type of exposure that occurs when the infection is spread through an object within the testing facility. The area must be cleaned and covered. Droplet exposure occurs when a fluid from the patient is dropped from the collection site.

**120. What is the purpose of wearing gloves in the laboratory setting?**

A. It protects the patient.

B. It protects the technician.

C. Both A and B

D. Neither A nor B

Answer: C. Both A and B

Explanation:  Gloves are worn to not only protect the patient while obtaining a sample, but to also protect the technician from exposure.

**121. The phlebotomy technician should wash his or her hands:**

A. Before and after contact with patients.

B. Before and after using the bathroom.

C. Prior to leaving the laboratory.

D. All of the above.

Answer: D. All of the above

Explanation: Hand washing must occur before and after each contact with a patient, in between providing a single patient with different tests, when the hands are contaminated with matter, before and after using the bathroom facility, prior to leaving the lab, before and after taking a break for lunch, and before using the protective gloves and after they are removed.

**122. If a person is requesting patient information, and he or she is not from a medical facility, what is required before the information is released?**

A. The patient must give consent in writing.
B. The patient must give oral consent.
C. The person requesting information must give consent in writing.
D. The person requesting information must give oral consent.

Answer: A. The patient must give consent in writing.

Explanation: Anyone who is requesting information about the patient must properly identify themselves. If the person who is requesting the information is from a medical facility, his or her identity must be confirmed. If a person requesting information is not from a medical facility, his or her name must be on the HIPAA form filled out by the patient in order to receive any information regarding the patient in question.

**123. Of the following statements, which is NOT accurate regarding HIPAA guidelines?**

    A. When using electronic devices for communication regarding a patient's care, the safety standards under the HIPAA regulations must be met.

    B. The HIPAA form provided by the patient must be kept up-to-date.

    C. Any changes within the policy must be discussed with the physician.

    D. Any paperwork or electronic records that have identifying patient information must be protected with the appropriate methods.

Answer: C. Any changes within the policy must be discussed with the physician.

Explanation: Any changes within the policy must be discussed with the patient, and a new form should be generated accordingly.

**124. If contact is made with exposed material, the area must be:**

    A. Washed with warm soapy water.

    B. Washed with a cleansing solution that meets OSHA standards.

    C. Washed with an antiseptic, such as alcohol.

    D. Washed with a clean cloth.

Answer: B. Washed with a cleansing solution that meets OSHA standards.

Explanation: If contact is made with the exposed material, the proper method of precaution must be used. The area that made contact with the infectious material must be washed with a cleansing solution that meets the standards by OSHA.

**125. What factors contribute to a strong immune system?**

    A.  Good eating habits.
    B.  Up-to-date immunizations.
    C.  Stress reduction.
    D.  All of the above.

Answer: D. All of the above.

Explanation: Those working within the facility must create a strong immune system to fight off the risk of infection. They must have up-to-date immunizations, ensure good eating and sleep habits, and practice stress reduction techniques.

**126. When a biohazard incident occurs within the laboratory, the phlebotomy technician must fill out the proper paperwork according to:**

    A.  OSHA standards
    B.  The facility's standards
    C.  Both A and B
    D.  Neither A nor B

Answer: C. Both A and B

Explanation: When a biohazard incident occurs within the laboratory, the phlebotomy technician must fill out the proper paperwork according to OSHA and the facility's standards. On the form, items listed will include the type of incident, the details of the incident, and people involved in the incident. This form will be copied and kept on file by the laboratory supervisor.

**127. What is the purpose of gloves in the laboratory setting?**

A. They protect the physician from infection transmission.
B. They stop the spread of many forms of contamination.
C. They protect the patient when the technician is taking the specimen.
D. All of the above

Answer: C. They protect the patient when the technician is taking the specimen.

Explanation: Gloves are worn to not only protect the patient while obtaining a sample, but to also protect the technician from exposure. The gloves worn by the technician provide a protective barrier when touching different materials and body parts involved within the testing process. They also stop the spread of cross contamination during the use of different items. Lastly, the gloves protect the patient from transmission of infection when touching the patient and taking the sample from areas where open skin may be present.

**128. Which of the following is NOT a form of protective facial equipment?**

A. Masks
B. Goggles
C. Protective eyewear
D. Gown

Answer: D. Gown

Explanation: Facial equipment is designed to protect workers from infection material in the form of droplets or airborne matter. This equipment includes facial masks, goggles, and protective eyewear. The mask worn will protect the patient and/or phlebotomy technician from exposure to small drops of fluid, which can travel a great distance.

**129. The phlebotomy technician should wash his or her hands:**

    A.  Before using the bathroom facility.
    B.  After using the bathroom facility
    C.  Both A and B
    D.  Neither A nor B

Answer: Both A and B

Explanation: Hand washing must occur before and after each contact with a patient, and before and after using the bathroom facility.

**130. What is the correct amount of hand sanitizer to use?**

    A.  ½ a teaspoon
    B.  1 teaspoon
    C.  2 teaspoons
    D.  1 Tablespoon

Answer: B. 1 teaspoon

Explanation: The sanitizer used within a lab is of medical grade, and the phlebotomy technician should use approximately one teaspoon of the sanitizer.

## 131. Why is proper hand washing important in the laboratory setting?

A. Because the hands are commonly exposed to bacteria.
B. Because the hands come in contact with blood often.
C. Because the hands often have open sores.
D. Because the patient often shakes hands with the technician.

Answer: A. Because the hands are commonly exposed to bacteria.

Explanation: Hand washing with the proper technique is considered vital because the hands are commonly exposed to bacteria. When bacteria from an infectious person are left on the hands, the infection can spread from the hands and into the body through open wounds or nail beds. In addition, touching another area of your body or the patient's body prior to removing the bacteria will cause spread and raise the risk of infection.

## 132. The first aid station present in the laboratory or healthcare facility must be:

A. Readily available to the technician.
B. Within 20 feet of the technician.
C. Within 20 yards of the technician.
D. Somewhere within the building.

Answer: A. Readily available to the technician.

Explanation: The first aid station present in the facility must be readily available to the technician. This means the station must be nearby, and set up properly in order to provide the right first aid care to the patient.

**133. The items found within the first aid box must be:**

A. Inspected on a regular basis.
B. In good condition.
C. Readily available.
D. All of the above.

Answer: D. All of the above.

Explanation: The items found within the first aid box must be in good condition and inspected on a regular basis. In addition, the box must contain the appropriate amount of materials, as specified by the board. When the materials within the box are used, new items should replace them.

**134. What should NOT be contained in the first aid kit/box?**

A. Medications
B. Wound care supplies
C. Gloves
D. Cardiopulmonary resuscitation mask

Answer: A. Medications

Explanation: Other than the regular contents for the first aid box, the box should also contain gloves of varying sizes to be used when providing first aid treatment. Medication should not be kept in the box where the first aid materials are stored. Finally, the box of materials should also contain a cardiopulmonary resuscitation (CPR) mask.

**135. A phlebotomy technician is assisting a patient who fell in the laboratory. The patient received a large 2-inch gash on his forehead. What should the technician do first?**

    A. Provide basic first aid to the patient.
    B. Call for help.
    C. Administer stitches.
    D. Leave to go get the supervisor.

Answer: A. Provide basic first aid to the patient.

Explanation: When providing first aid to the patient, the injured area must be examined in order to determine the best method of treatment. The materials needed for the treatment can be obtained from the box, so treatment then can be given to the patient. In certain cases, such as the need for stiches, bleeding must be treated, and then, the technician should call for assistance per facility protocol.

**136. How often is cardiopulmonary resuscitation (CPR) training necessary?**

    A. Every 6 months
    B. Every year
    C. Every 2 years
    D. Every 3 years

Answer: C. Every 2 years

Explanation: Many healthcare facilities and laboratories recommend that all phlebotomy technicians have an up-to-date certification in CPR in order to practice within the field. The CPR will need to be obtained prior to employment, and then it must be renewed every two years in order to ensure it is valid.

**137. When CPR certification is granted, the certificate must be placed:**

    A. In a location where it is visible to the patients.
    B. In a location where it is visible to other healthcare workers.
    C. Both A and B
    D. Neither A nor B

Answer: C. Both A and B

Explanation: In a location that makes it viable to the patient and other healthcare workers. When providing CPR to a patient, the use of the mask that is available within the first aid box must always be applied.

**138. What is the purpose of the CPR mask during resuscitation?**

    A. To provide an effective barrier between the patient and healthcare worker.
    B. To protect the patient.
    C. To protect the healthcare worker.
    D. All of the above.

Answer: D. All of the above.

Explanation: When CPR certification is granted, the certificate must be placed in a location that makes it viable to the patient and other healthcare workers. When providing CPR to a patient, the use of the mask that is available within the first aid box must always be applied. This mask will ensure that both the healthcare worker and the patient are protected during the CPR process, as it works to create an effective barrier between the two when providing the patient will oxygen.

**139. The process of CPR requires the use of the steps C-A-B. What does the C abbreviate?**

    A. Circulation
    B. Cardiac
    C. Coronary
    D. Critical

Answer: A. Circulation

Explanation: The process of CPR requires the proper use of steps C-A-B. Circulation (C) involves the presence of proper circulation. This involves learning how to properly place the patient so that circulation is not affected during the session of CPR. Circulation is achieved through 30 chest compressions.

**140. When attending a patient who needs CPR, how many rescue breaths are given initially?**

    A. One
    B. Two
    C. Three
    D. Four

Answer: B. Two

Explanation: In order to properly stabilize the patient through the process of CPR, you need to breathe for the patient. First, you must give the patient two rescue breaths, which are needed in order to see if the chest rises in the patient. If the chest does not rise after the rescue breathes are provided, the patient must be given another set of chest compressions, followed by two more rescue breaths. In between cycles, the patient's breathing and heartbeat should be assessed.

**141. When providing CPR, if someone arrives prior to the patient being stabilized, they should be instructed to:**

    A.  Assist with rescue breathing.
    B.  Assist with chest compressions.
    C.  Call for help.
    D.  Both A and B

Answer: C. Call for help.

Explanation: Once another person is present to look after the patient, and the patient is stabilized, the call to the right emergency professionals can be made. If someone arrives prior to the patient become stabilized, they should be instructed to call for help while you continue with the CPR process.

**142. What type of transmission occurs when a fluid from the patient is dropped from the collection site?**

    A.  Contact transmission
    B.  Droplet transmission
    C.  Indirect contact transmission
    D.  Airborne transmission

Answer: D. Airborne transmission

Explanation: This occurs when a fluid from the patient is dropped from the collection site. If droplet exposure occurs, the area must be evacuated if the fluid is infectious. When droplet exposure occurs, and no known infection is present, a specialized solution must be applied to the area. In addition, the fluid must be cleaned from the area in order for the space to be safe again.

**143. What type of transmission is contact with an infectious material?**

    A.  Contact transmission
    B.  Airborne transmission
    C.  Direct transmission
    D.  Indirect transmission

Answer: A. Contact transmission

Explanation: If contact is made with the exposed material, the proper method of precaution must be used. The area that made contact with the infectious material must be washed with a cleansing solution that meets the standards by OSHA.

**144. Standards created to obtain accurate testing results from the sample collected by the patient are called:**

A. Quality assurance

B. Quality control

C. Risk management

D. Total quality management

Answer: B. Quality control

Explanation: Quality control (QC) was created to obtain accurate testing results from the sample collected by the patient.

**145. What contains a list of policies and procedures set in place to reduce health risks to both the patient and the technician?**

    A.  Quality assurance
    B.  Quality control
    C.  Total quality management
    D.  Risk management

Answer: D. Risk management

Explanation: Risk management (RM) contains a list of policies and procedures set in place to reduce health risks to both the patient and the technician.

**146. Precaution used in the event of an occupational exposure should be based upon:**

    A.  The type of bodily fluid
    B.  The type of exposure
    C.  The type of tissue or organ
    D.  The type of HIV cells

Answer: B. The type of exposure

Explanation: The exposure that occurs must be labeled with the correct level of risk present. Those working within the facility must also be classified in different according to individual risk. For example, those working directly with the patient are considered to be of the highest risk to exposure, while those who provide clerical duties are considered the lowest exposure risk.

**147. Laboratories will have random inspections completed to ensure that they are:**

A. Testing with waived methods.
B. Testing with non-waived methods.
C. Testing with OSHA methods.
D. Testing with CLIM methods.

Answer: A. Testing with waived methods.

Explanation: Laboratories will have random inspections completed to ensure that they are only testing with waived testing methods.

**148. Proficiency testing ensures that all people collecting the samples are following the guidelines and the testing requirements in order to:**

A. Provide the most accurate results.
B. Provide the least accurate results.
C. Perform the quality control.
D. Perform the quality assurance.

Answer: A. Provide the most accurate results.

Explanation: Through proficiency testing, all people collecting the samples are following the guidelines, and the testing requirements provide the most accurate results.

**149. By performing the quality control testing process, the facility:**

A. Meets the standards required by the quality assurance plan and CLIA guidelines.
B. Meets the standards required by the quality control plan and CLIM guidelines.
C. Meets the standards required by the quality control detector and OSHA guidelines.
D. Meets the standards required by the quality control device and CLIA guidelines.

Answer: A. Meets the standards required by the quality assurance plan and CLIA guidelines.

Explanation: By performing the quality control testing process, the facility meets the standards required by the quality assurance plan and CLIA guidelines. There are now testing devices with built-in quality control detectors.

**150. Stools are generally collected within a two-tube test, and each tube should be filled:**

A. At least 14 hours apart from the other.
B. At least one day apart from the other.
C. At least two days apart from the other.
D. At least three days apart from the other.

Explanation: The stools are generally collected within a two-tube test, and each tube should be filled at least one day apart from the other. No more than two tubes should be used for the patient testing. When a stool sample is needed from a pediatric patient, a swab sample of the stool is taken.

# Exclusive Trivium Test Tips

Here at Trivium Test Prep, we strive to offer you the exemplary test tools that help you pass your exam the first time. This book includes an overview of important concepts, example questions throughout the text, and practice test questions. But we know that learning how to successfully take a test can be just as important as learning the content being tested. In addition to excelling on the CPT, we want to give you the solutions you need to be successful every time you take a test. Our study strategies, preparation pointers, and test tips will help you succeed as you take the CPT and any test in the future!

## Study Strategies

1.  Spread out your studying. By taking the time to study a little bit every day, you strengthen your understanding of the testing material, so it's easier to recall that information on the day of the test. Our study guides make this easy by breaking up the concepts into sections with example practice questions, so you can test your knowledge as you read.

2.  Create a study calendar. The sections of our book make it easy to review and practice with example questions on a schedule. Decide to read a specific number of pages or complete a number of practice questions every day. Breaking up all of the information in this way can make studying less overwhelming and more manageable.

3.  Set measurable goals and motivational rewards. Follow your study calendar and reward yourself for completing reading, example questions, and practice problems and tests. You could take yourself out after a productive week of studying or watch a favorite show after reading a chapter. Treating yourself to rewards is a great way to stay motivated.

4.  Use your current knowledge to understand new, unfamiliar concepts. When you learn something new, think about how it relates to something you know really well. Making connections between new ideas and your existing understanding can simplify the learning process and make the new information easier to remember.

5.  Make learning interesting! If one aspect of a topic is interesting to you, it can make an entire concept easier to remember. Stay engaged and think about how concepts covered on the exam can affect the things you're interested in. The sidebars throughout the text offer additional information that could make ideas easier to recall.

6.  Find a study environment that works for you. For some people, absolute silence in a library results in the most effective study session, while others need the background noise of a coffee shop to fuel productive studying. There are many websites that generate white noise and recreate the sounds of different environments for studying. Figure out what distracts you and what engages you and plan accordingly.

7.  Take practice tests in an environment that reflects the exam setting. While it's important to be as comfortable as possible when you study, practicing taking the test exactly as you'll take it on test day will make you more prepared for the actual exam. If your test starts on a Saturday morning, take your practice test on a Saturday

morning. If you have access, try to find an empty classroom that has desks like the desks at testing center. The more closely you can mimic the testing center, the more prepared you'll feel on test day.

8. Study hard for the test in the days before the exam, but take it easy the night before and do something relaxing rather than studying and cramming. This will help decrease anxiety, allow you to get a better night's sleep, and be more mentally fresh during the big exam. Watch a light-hearted movie, read a favorite book, or take a walk, for example.

## Preparation Pointers

1. Preparation is key! Don't wait until the day of your exam to gather your pencils, calculator, identification materials, or admission tickets. Check the requirements of the exam as soon as possible. Some tests require materials that may take more time to obtain, such as a passport-style photo, so be sure that you have plenty of time to collect everything. The night before the exam, lay out everything you'll need, so it's all ready to go on test day! We recommend at least two forms of ID, your admission ticket or confirmation, pencils, a high protein, compact snack, bottled water, and any necessary medications. Some testing centers will require you to put all of your supplies in a clear plastic bag. If you're prepared, you will be less stressed the morning of, and less likely to forget anything important.

2. If you're taking a pencil-and-paper exam, test your erasers on paper. Some erasers leave big, dark stains on paper instead of rubbing out pencil marks. Make sure your erasers work for you and the pencils you plan to use.

3. Make sure you give yourself your usual amount of sleep, preferably at least 7 – 8 hours. You may find you need even more sleep. Pay attention to how much you sleep in the days before the exam, and how many hours it takes for you to feel refreshed. This will allow you to be as sharp as possible during the test and make fewer simple mistakes.

4. Make sure to make transportation arrangements ahead of time, and have a backup plan in case your ride falls through. You don't want to be stressing about how you're going to get to the testing center the morning of the exam.

5. Many testing locations keep their air conditioners on high. You want to remember to bring a sweater or jacket in case the test center is too cold, as you never know how hot or cold the testing location could be. Remember, while you can always adjust for heat by removing layers, if you're cold, you're cold.

## Test Tips

1. Go with your gut when choosing an answer. Statistically, the answer that comes to mind first is often the right one. This is assuming you studied the material, of course, which we hope you have done if you've read through one of our books!

2. For true or false questions: if you genuinely don't know the answer, mark it true. In most tests, there are typically more true answers than false answers.

3. For multiple-choice questions, read ALL the answer choices before marking an answer, even if you think you know the answer when you come across it. You may find your original "right" answer isn't necessarily the best option.

4. Look for key words: in multiple choice exams, particularly those that require you to read through a text, the questions typically contain key words. These key words can help the test taker choose the correct answer or confuse you if you don't recognize them. Common keywords are: *most, during, after, initially,* and *first.* Be sure you identify them before you read the available answers. Identifying the key words makes a huge difference in your chances of passing the test.

5. Narrow answers down by using the process of elimination: after you understand the question, read each answer. If you don't know the answer right away, use the process of elimination to narrow down the answer choices. It is easy to identify at least one answer that isn't correct. Continue to narrow down the choices before choosing the answer you believe best fits the question. By following this process, you increase your chances of selecting the correct answer.

6. Don't worry if others finish before or after you. Go at your own pace, and focus on the test in front of you.

7. Relax. With our help, we know you'll be ready to conquer the CPT. You've studied and worked hard!

Keep in mind that every individual takes tests differently, so strategies that might work for you may not work for someone else. You know yourself best and are the best person to determine which of these tips and strategies will benefit your studying and test taking. Best of luck as you study, test, and work toward your future!

Made in the
USA
Columbia, SC